Drugs of Choice

2021

Selected 2020 Articles from
The Medical Letter on Drugs and Therapeutics®

Published by

The Medical Letter, Inc.
145 Huguenot St.
New Rochelle, New York 10801-7537

800-211-2769
914-235-0500
Fax 914-632-1733
www.medicalletter.org

22nd Edition

The Medical Letter Inc.
145 Huguenot St., Ste. 312
New Rochelle, New York 10801-7537

Contents

Tables

Postmenopausal Osteoporosis

Introduction

The Medical Letter, Inc. is a nonprofit organization that publishes critical appraisals of new prescription drugs and comparative reviews of drugs for common diseases in its newsletter, *The Medical Letter on Drugs and Therapeutics*. It is committed to providing objective, practical, and timely information on drugs and treatments of common diseases to help readers make the best decisions for their patients—without the influence of the pharmaceutical industry. The Medical Letter is supported by its readers, and does not receive any commercial support or accept advertising in any of its publications.

Many of our readers know that pharmaceutical companies and their representatives often exaggerate the therapeutic effects and understate the adverse effects of their products, but busy practitioners have neither the time nor the resources to check the accuracy of the manufacturers' claims. Our publication is intended specifically to meet the needs of busy healthcare professionals who want unbiased, reliable, and timely drug information. Our editorial process is designed to ensure that the information we provide represents an unbiased consensus of medical experts.

The editorial process used for *The Medical Letter on Drugs and Therapeutics* relies on a consensus of experts to develop prescribing recommendations. The first draft of an article is prepared by one of our in-house or contributing editors or by an outside expert. This initial draft is edited and sent to our Contributing Editors, to 10-20 other reviewers who have clinical and/or experimental experience with the drug or type of drug or disease under review, to the FDA, and to the first and last authors of all the articles cited in the text. Many critical observations, suggestions, and questions are received from the reviewers and are incorporated into the article during the revision process. Further communication as needed is followed by fact checking and editing to make sure the final appraisal is not only accurate, but also easy to read.

DRUGS FOR
ADHD

Original publication date — January 2020

Attention-deficit/hyperactivity disorder (ADHD) is a chronic neuro-developmental disorder that has been diagnosed in up to 10% of school-age children in the US and frequently persists into adulthood.[1,2] A study in a large Danish cohort found that ADHD was associated with higher mortality rates in children, adolescents, and adults, mainly due to accidents.[3] Pharmacologic treatment of ADHD in children has been reported to decrease the risk of substance abuse in adolescents, and use of ADHD medications in adults has been associated with a reduced risk of serious traffic accidents and criminal behavior.[4-6] Drugs approved by the FDA for treatment of ADHD are listed in Table 1.

BEHAVIORAL THERAPIES

Parent Training in Behavior Management (PTBM) and/or behavioral classroom interventions are recommended by the American Academy of Pediatrics for first-line treatment of preschool-age children with ADHD. Medication is the first-line therapy for children 6-12 years old and adolescents, but family- and school-based training and behavioral therapies are strongly recommended as an adjunct to medication. Children receiving behavioral therapy may respond to lower doses of ADHD drugs than those receiving medication alone.[7,8]

Summary: Drugs for ADHD
Behavioral Therapies
► Parent Training in Behavior Management (PTBM) and/or behavioral classroom interventions are the first line of treatment for preschool-age children and are strongly recommended as an adjunct to medication in school-age children and adolescents.
Stimulants
► Stimulants, which are schedule II controlled substances, are the drugs of choice for treatment of ADHD in school-age children, adolescents, and adults. Some patients may respond better to amphetamines than to methylphenidate and vice versa.
► Use of long-acting formulations, which generally contain both immediate- and extended-release components, has become standard clinical practice. A short-acting formulation may be used in addition to improve symptom control early in the morning or to prolong the duration of action in the afternoon.
► Common adverse effects include decreased appetite, abdominal pain, headache, and sleep disturbances. Psychotic symptoms, cardiovascular events, and abuse and dependence can occur.
► Long-term use has been associated with reduced adult height.
Nonstimulants
► The alpha$_2$-agonists clonidine and guanfacine and the selective norepinephrine reuptake inhibitor atomoxetine can reduce ADHD symptoms, but they are less effective than stimulants. They can be used in combination with stimulants or when stimulants are contraindicated, ineffective, or not tolerated.
► They are not controlled substances.
► Clonidine and guanfacine can cause somnolence, dizziness, and hypotension.
► Atomoxetine can cause somnolence, nausea, vomiting, increases in heart rate and blood pressure, and growth delays. An increased risk of suicidal thoughts has been reported.

STIMULANTS

All of the stimulants used for treatment of ADHD are classified as schedule II controlled substances (highest potential for abuse; recognized medical use).

METHYLPHENIDATE — Methylphenidate has been shown to be effective in improving ADHD symptoms in both children and adults.

Short-acting methylphenidate formulations (*Ritalin*, and others) are rapidly absorbed; effects on behavior can be seen within 30-60 minutes of administration and persist for 3-5 hours. Because of their short duration of action, mid-day dosing during school is usually required. Short-acting formulations of methylphenidate are sometimes used in addition to longer-acting formulations to improve symptom control early in the morning or to prolong duration and smooth withdrawal in the late afternoon.

Intermediate-acting methylphenidate formulations have a slower onset of action than short-acting formulations and a duration of action of up to 8 hours. These drugs may be better tolerated by children who are sensitive to stimulant side effects, but they are highly variable in duration and efficacy.

Long-acting methylphenidate formulations dosed once daily have become the standard of care.[9] Most contain a combination of immediate-release and delayed- or extended-release components. Their onset of action is generally within 20-60 minutes; the duration of action varies from 8 to 16 hours. Long-acting methylphenidate formulations that can be used in patients who are unable to swallow a tablet or capsule include capsules that can be opened and sprinkled on food (*Focalin XR*, and others), a chewable tablet *(Quillichew ER)*,[10] an orally disintegrating tablet *(Cotempla XR-ODT)*,[11] an oral suspension *(Quillivant XR)*,[12] and a transdermal patch *(Daytrana)*.[13] The transdermal patch should be applied 2 hours before an effect is needed; the delay in its onset of action can be a disadvantage when getting children ready for school in the morning.

Jornay PM, a delayed- and extended-release capsule formulation that is taken at night, offers an alternative for patients who have disruptive symptoms upon waking; the microbeads contained in the capsules are coated with a delayed-release outer layer that prevents release of methylphenidate for about 8-10 hours after ingestion and with an extended-release inner layer that gradually releases the drug throughout the day.[14]

AMPHETAMINES — Amphetamines generally have been as effective as methylphenidate in improving ADHD symptoms in children

3

Table 1. Some Drugs for ADHD

Drug	Some Available Formulations	Duration of Action
Methylphenidate Stimulants		
Dexmethylphenidate		
Short-Acting − generic Focalin (Novartis)	2.5, 5, 10 mg tabs	5-6 h
Long-Acting − generic Focalin XR	5, 10, 15, 20, 25, 30, 35, 40 mg ER caps[4,5]	12 h
Methylphenidate		
Short-Acting − generic	5, 10, 20 mg tabs and chewable tabs; 5 mg/5 mL, 10 mg/5 mL soln	3-5 h
Ritalin (Novartis)	5, 10, 20 mg tabs	
Methylin Oral Solution (Shionogi)	5 mg/5 mL, 10 mg/5 mL soln[6]	
Intermediate-Acting − generic	10, 20 mg ER tabs[7]	8 h
Long-Acting − Adhansia XR[8] (Adlon)	25, 35, 45, 55, 70, 85 mg ER caps[5,9]	13-16 h
Aptensio XR[8] (Rhodes)	10, 15, 20, 30, 40, 50, 60 mg ER caps[5,10]	12 h
Concerta (Janssen) generic	18, 27, 36, 54 mg ER tabs[7,11]	10-12 h
Cotempla XR-ODT[8] (Neos)	8.6, 17.3, 25.9 mg ER ODT[13,14]	12 h
Daytrana (Noven)	10, 15, 20, 30 mg ER transdermal patches[16]	10-12 h

ER = extended-release; ODT = orally disintegrating tablets; SR = sustained-release
1. For children ≥6 years old.
2. Approximate WAC for 30 days' treatment at the lowest initial pediatric dosage. WAC = wholesaler acquisition cost or manufacturer's published price to wholesalers; WAC represents a published catalogue or list price and may not represent an actual transactional price. Source: AnalySource® Monthly. January 5, 2020. Reprinted with permission by First Databank, Inc. All rights reserved. ©2020. www.fdbhealth.com/policies/drug-pricing-policy.
3. ND Volkow and JM Swanson. N Engl J Med 2013; 369:1935.
4. Contains 50% immediate-release beads and 50% enteric-coated, delayed-release beads.
5. The contents of the capsule may be sprinkled on a small amount of soft food (e.g., applesauce).
6. Available in bottles containing 500 mL.
7. Must be swallowed whole, not crushed or chewed.
8. Alcohol consumption may increase the rate of release of methylphenidate and should be avoided.
9. Contains 20% immediate-release and 80% controlled-release particles.

Pediatric Dosage[1] Initial/Maximum	Adult Dosage Initial/Maximum	Cost[2]
2.5 mg bid/10 mg bid	2.5 mg bid/10 mg bid[3]	$12.60
		38.00
5 mg qAM/30 mg qAM	10 mg qAM/40 mg qAM	120.90
		380.50

5 mg bid/60 mg divided bid
  or tid
	10 mg bid/60 mg divided bid
	  or tid
		15.30

		39.40
		21.00
10 mg qAM/60 mg qAM	10 mg qAM/60 mg qAM	90.00
25 mg qAM/85 mg qAM	25 mg qAM/100 mg qAM	299.40
10 mg qAM/60 mg qAM	10 mg qAM/60 mg qAM	250.10
18 mg qAM/54-72 mg qAM[12]	18 or 36 mg qAM/72 mg qAM	347.60
		169.80
17.3 mg qAM/51.8 mg qAM	See footnote 15	420.00

10 mg patch on 9 hrs, off
  15 hrs/30 mg patch on 9 hrs,
  off 15 hrs[17]
	See footnote 15	396.30

10. Contains 40% immediate-release and 60% controlled-release particles.
11. Tablets contain 20% of the dose for immediate-release and 80% for extended-release over 6-7 hours.
12. The maximum recommended daily dose is 54 mg for children 6-12 years old and 72 mg for adolescents 13-17 years old.
13. Contains 25% immediate-release and 75% extended-release particles. Doses of 8.6, 17.3, and 25.9 mg are equivalent to 10, 20, and 30 mg, respectively, of methylphenidate hydrochloride.
14. The tablet should be placed on the tongue and swallowed after it disintegrates. It should not be crushed or chewed.
15. FDA-approved based on studies in children and adolescents.
16. *Daytrana* is supplied in a sealed tray or outer pouch containing 30 patches in individual pouches.
17. The patch should be applied 2 hours before an effect is needed. Effects will last for up to 3 hours after the patch is removed. The patch can be removed before 9 hours if a shorter duration of action is desired.

Continued on next page

Table 1. Some Drugs for ADHD (continued)

Drug	Some Available Formulations	Duration of Action
Methylphenidate Stimulants (continued)		
Intermediate-Acting – (continued)		
Jornay PM[8] (Ironshore)	20, 40, 60, 80, 100 mg ER caps[5,18]	7-12 h[19]
methylphenidate CD – generic[8]	10, 20, 30, 40, 50, 60 mg ER caps[5,20]	8-12 h
QuilliChew ER[8] (Tris)	20, 30, 40 mg ER chewable tabs[21]	12 h
Quillivant XR[8] (Tris)	25 mg/5 mL ER susp[22,23]	12 h
Ritalin LA (Novartis)[24] generic	10, 20, 30, 40 mg ER caps[4,5]	8-12 h
Amphetamine Stimulants[25]		
Amphetamine		
Adzenys ER (Neos)	1.25 mg/mL ER susp[26,27]	10-12 h
Adzenys XR-ODT	3.1, 6.3, 9.4, 12.5, 15.7, 18.8 mg ER ODT[14,26,27]	10-12 h
Dyanavel XR (Tris)	2.5 mg/mL ER susp[29]	13 h
Racemic amphetamine sulfate		
Evekeo[30] (Arbor)	5, 10 mg tabs	10 h[31]
Evekeo ODT	5, 10, 15, 20 mg ODT[14]	10 h[31]
Mixed amphetamine salts		
Short-Acting[30] – generic *Adderall* (Teva)	5, 7.5, 10, 12.5, 15, 20, 30 mg tabs	4-6 h

ER = extended-release; ODT = orally disintegrating tablets; SR = sustained-release
18. Contains delayed-release beads (prevent release of methylphenidate for 8-10 hours) and extended-release beads.
19. From onset of action.
20. Contains 30% immediate-release and 70% delayed-release beads.
21. Contains 30% immediate-release and 70% extended-release particles.
22. Contains 20% immediate-release and 80% extended-release particles.
23. Must be reconstituted before administration and is stable for up to 4 months. It is available in bottles containing 60, 120, 150, or 180 mL.
24. FDA-approved only for use in children 6-12 years old.
25. Alkalinizing agents can increase serum concentrations of amphetamines and acidifying agents can decrease them.

Pediatric Dosage[1] Initial/Maximum	Adult Dosage Initial/Maximum	Cost[2]
20 mg qPM/100 mg qPM	20 mg qPM/100 mg qPM	$370.00
20 mg qAM/60 mg qAM	20 mg qAM/80 mg qAM	117.90
20 mg qAM/60 mg qAM	20 mg qAM/60 mg qAM	351.70
20 mg qAM/60 mg qAM	20 mg qAM/60 mg qAM	310.50
10-20 mg qAM/60 mg qAM	10-20 mg qAM/60 mg qAM[3]	298.60 198.30
6.3 mg qAM/12.5-18.8 mg qAM[28]	12.5 mg qAM/12.5 mg qAM	226.30
6.3 mg qAM/18.8 mg qAM[28]	12.5 mg qAM/12.5 mg qAM	360.00
2.5-5 mg qAM/20 mg qAM	2.5-5 mg qAM/20 mg qAM	79.50
5 mg qAM or bid[32]/40 mg divided bid	See footnote 15	200.30
5 mg qAM or bid/40 mg divided bid	See footnote 15	200.30
5 mg qAM or bid[32]/40 mg divided bid	5 mg bid/60 mg divided bid[3]	17.40 224.60

26. Contains approximately 50% immediate-release and 50% delayed-release particles.
27. Doses of 3.1, 6.3, 9.4, 12.5, 15.7, and 18.8 mg are equivalent to 5, 10, 15, 20, 25, and 30 mg, respectively of *Adderall XR*.
28. The maximum recommended daily dose is 18.8 mg for children 6-12 years old and 12.5 mg for adolescents 13-17 years old.
29. 2.5 mg of amphetamine base is equivalent to 4 mg of mixed amphetamine salts products. Available in bottles containing 464 mL.
30. FDA-approved for use in children ≥3 years old.
31. AC Childress et al. J Child Adolesc Psychopharmacol 2015; 25:402.
32. Initial dosage for children 3-5 years old is 2.5 mg once daily.

Continued on next page

Drug	Some Available Formulations	Duration of Action
Table 1. Some Drugs for ADHD (continued)		
Amphetamine Stimulants[25] (continued)		
Mixed amphetamine salts (continued)		
Long-Acting – generic	5, 10, 15, 20, 25, 30 mg ER caps[5]	10-12 h
Adderall XR (Shire)		
Mydayis (Shire)[34]	12.5, 25, 37.5, 50 mg ER caps[5,35]	16 h
Dextroamphetamines		
Short-Acting[30] – generic	5, 10 mg tabs; 5 mg/5 mL soln	4-6 h
Zenzedi (Arbor)	2.5, 5, 7.5, 10, 15, 20, 30 mg tabs	
ProCentra (Independence)	5 mg/5 mL soln[37]	
Long-Acting – generic	5, 10, 15 mg SR caps[7]	8-12 h
Dexedrine Spansules (Impax/Amneal)		
Lisdexamfetamine dimesylate		
Vyvanse (Shire)	10, 20, 30, 40, 50, 60, 70 mg caps[5]; 10, 20, 30, 40, 50, 60 mg chewable tabs	13-14 h[38]
Nonstimulants		
Guanfacine extended-release – generic	1, 2, 3, 4 mg ER tabs[7]	8-24 h[38]
Intuniv (Shire)		
Clonidine extended-release – generic	0.1 mg ER tabs[7]	12 h[38]
Kapvay (Concordia)		

ER = extended-release; ODT = orally disintegrating tablets; SR = sustained-release
33. Recommended dosage in patients with severe renal impairment (GFR 15 to <30 mL/min/1.73 m²) is 5 mg qAM for children (max 20 mg once/day in children 6-12 years old) and 15 mg qAM for adults. Not recommended in patients with end-stage renal disease.
34. FDA-approved only for patients ≥13 years old.
35. Contains immediate-release beads, and 2 types of delayed-release beads that release amphetamine at pH 5.5 and at pH 7.0.
36. The maximum recommended dosage in patients with severe renal impairment (GFR 15 to <30 mL/min/1.73 m²) is 12.5 mg/day for children and 15 mg/day for adults. Not recommended in patients with end-stage renal disease.

Pediatric Dosage[1] Initial/Maximum	Adult Dosage Initial/Maximum	Cost[2]
10 mg qAM/30 mg qAM[33]	20 mg qAM/30 mg qAM[33]	$78.60 213.70
12.5 mg qAM/25 mg qAM[36]	12.5 mg qAM/50 mg qAM[36]	278.80
5 mg qAM or bid[32]/40 mg divided bid	5 mg bid/60 mg divided bid[3]	27.00 214.10 253.70
5 mg qAM or bid/60 mg qAM or divided bid	5 mg qAM or bid/60 mg qAM or divided bid[3]	171.60 703.20
30 mg qAM/70 mg qAM[39]	30 mg qAM/70 mg qAM[39]	319.00
1 mg once daily/7 mg once daily[40,41]	See footnote 15	18.90 291.40
0.1 mg once daily at bedtime/ 0.4 mg divided bid[42]	See footnote 15	84.90 221.00

37. Available in bottles containing 473 mL.
38. According to the manufacturer.
39. The maximum recommended dosage in patients with severe renal impairment (GFR 15 to <30 mL/min/1.73 m²) is 50 mg/day; in patients with end-stage renal disease it is 30 mg/day.
40. Dose reductions for significant renal or hepatic impairment may be required.
41. Dosage adjustments are recommended with concomitant use of strong or moderate CYP3A4 inhibitors or CYP3A4 inducers.
42. Dosage of 0.4 mg/day is more likely to cause hypotension.

Continued on next page

Table 1. Some Drugs for ADHD (continued)		
Drug	**Some Available Formulations**	**Duration of Action**
Nonstimulants (continued)		
Atomoxetine – generic *Strattera* (Lilly)	10, 18, 25, 40, 60, 80, 100 mg caps	10-24 h

ER = extended-release; ODT = orally disintegrating tablets; SR = sustained-release
43. Dose for children weighing ≤70 kg. Children weighing >70 kg should use the adult dose.
44. Initial and target dosages should be reduced to 50% of normal in patients with moderate hepatic impairment (Child-Pugh B) and to 25% of normal in patients with severe hepatic impairment (Child-Pugh C).

and adults. They are available in short- and long-acting formulations. Long-acting formulations that are available for patients who have difficulty swallowing tablets or capsules include chewable tablets *(Vyvanse)*, orally disintegrating tablets *(Evekeo ODT; Adzenys XR-ODT)*,[15] liquids *(Adzenys ER; Dyanavel XR)*,[15,16] and capsules that can be opened and sprinkled on food.

Dextroamphetamine – The onset of action of short-acting dextroamphetamine *(Zenzedi, ProCentra,* and generics) occurs within 30-60 minutes of ingestion, and its duration of action is 4-6 hours. Twice-daily administration can extend the therapeutic effect throughout the school day but requires taking the second dose in school. Long-acting formulations *(Dexedrine Spansules,* and generics) have a duration of action of 8-12 hours and can be taken once daily.

Mixtures – Mixed amphetamine salts *(Adderall, Adderall XR* and generics; *Mydayis)* are available in short- and long-acting formulations. *Adderall XR*, which contains both immediate- and delayed-release beads, has a duration of action of 10 to 12 hours. *Mydayis,* which is formulated as capsules containing immediate-release beads and 2 types of delayed-release beads, has a duration of action of up to 16 hours.[17,18] It is FDA-approved only for use in patients ≥13 years old.

Pediatric Dosage[1] Initial/Maximum	Adult Dosage Initial/Maximum	Cost[2]
0.5 mg/kg/d in a single dose or divided bid/1.4 mg/kg/d in a single dose or divided bid (max 100 mg/d)[43-45]	40 mg once daily/100 mg once daily or divided bid[40]	$128.40[46] 429.60[46]

45. Patients who are CYP2D6 poor metabolizers or are taking strong CYP2D6 inhibitors should take the recommended initial dose; the dose should only be increased if it is well tolerated and symptoms fail to improve after 4 weeks of treatment.
46. Cost of 40-mg capsules.

Lisdexamfetamine – Lisdexamfetamine dimesylate *(Vyvanse)* is a prodrug of dextroamphetamine.[19] Its duration of action is 13-14 hours.[20] Lisdexamfetamine was directly compared with extended-release (ER) methylphenidate (*Concerta*, and generics) in two randomized, double-blind trials in adolescents with ADHD. In a 6-week forced-dose trial (n=549), lisdexamfetamine 70 mg/day was superior to ER methylphenidate 72 mg/day in improving ADHD rating scale scores. In an 8-week flexible-dose trial (n=464), there was no significant difference in efficacy between the drugs. In both trials, the incidence of adverse effects was slightly higher with lisdexamfetamine than with ER methylphenidate.[21]

DOSING OF STIMULANTS — Dosing requirements for stimulants are highly variable. Stimulants should be started at the lowest recommended dose, which can be increased every 7 days (in urgent cases every 3 days) until a substantial improvement in symptoms is achieved. Continued monitoring of effectiveness and tolerability at regular intervals is strongly recommended.

ADVERSE EFFECTS — The labels of all stimulants contain a boxed warning about the high risk of abuse and dependence associated with these drugs; patients should be monitored for signs of abuse. The most common short-term adverse effects of stimulants are appetite loss, abdominal pain, headache, and sleep disturbances. Tic disorders are common in patients receiving stimulants and have resulted in discontinuation of treatment, but a meta-analysis of controlled trials found that the risk of new-onset or worsening tics was similar in stimulant and placebo groups.[22] Some children, especially adolescents, say that stimulants make them feel less spontaneous and less comfortable in their social interactions.

In an observational study that followed 515 children with ADHD into early adulthood, long-term use of stimulants was associated with suppression of adult height; patients who consistently or inconsistently used stimulants were on average about 2.5 cm shorter as adults than those who reported negligible use.[23]

Tactile and visual hallucinations and other psychotic symptoms have occurred in patients taking stimulants. In a large cohort study, insurance claims data for 221,846 patients 13-25 years old with ADHD who started taking methylphenidate or an amphetamine were analyzed to identify those who received a new diagnosis of psychosis and a prescription for an antipsychotic medication. During a median follow-up of 4-5 months, the risk of new-onset psychosis was low, but it was about two times higher with amphetamines than with methylphenidate (237 episodes [0.21%] vs 106 episodes [0.10%]); the median time from starting a stimulant to having a psychotic episode was 128 days.[24] Stimulants should be used with caution in patients with a history of psychosis.

The labels of all stimulants contain a warning about a risk of cardio-vascular events and sudden death. These drugs usually cause only small increases in blood pressure and heart rate, but larger increases have been reported in 5-15% of patients; monitoring of heart rate and blood pressure is recommended.[25] Several large cohort studies have found no evidence that stimulants used to treat ADHD increase the risk of serious cardiovascular events in children or adults.[26-28] In the absence of a history (personal or familial) or clinical evidence of heart disease, an electro-cardiogram or a consultation with a cardiologist is not necessary before starting treatment with a stimulant.[29]

Stimulants rarely can cause priapism; boys and men should be instructed to seek immediate medical attention if it occurs.[30]

DRUG INTERACTIONS — Concurrent use of a CNS stimulant and a monoamine oxidase (MAO) inhibitor can result in hypertensive crisis and is contraindicated; stimulants should not be taken with or within 14 days after stopping an MAO inhibitor. Concomitant use of a CYP2D6 inhibitor may increase amphetamine serum concentrations.[31] Coadministration of an amphetamine and a serotonergic drug may increase the risk of serotonin syndrome.

Use of amphetamines with alkalinizing agents such as sodium bicarbonate, H2-receptor antagonists, or proton pump inhibitors can increase amphetamine serum concentrations. Coadministration with acidifying agents such as ascorbic acid can decrease their effects.

NONSTIMULANTS

ALPHA₂-AGONISTS — The alpha₂-adrenergic agonists guanfacine and clonidine were originally approved for treatment of hypertension, but they have been used off-label for many years for treatment of ADHD, particularly in children with tics.[32] ER formulations of both drugs have been approved by the FDA for use as monotherapy and as an adjunct to a stimulant in children 6-17 years old with ADHD. Neither is a controlled substance.

In pharmacokinetic studies, multiple 4-mg doses of **ER guanfacine** (*Intuniv,* and generics) produced higher serum concentrations of the drug in children 6-12 years old than in those 13-17 years old. ER guanfacine has been shown to be modestly more effective than placebo in producing improvement on ADHD rating scales.[33] Treatment with **ER clonidine** (*Kapvay*, and generics) has also resulted in modest improvements in inattention, hyperactivity, and impulsivity compared to placebo. Children treated with both a stimulant and clonidine have shown significantly greater improvement in ADHD symptoms than those treated with a stimulant alone.[34]

Adverse Effects – Adverse effects of alpha$_2$-agonists include somnolence, dry mouth, dizziness, headache, bradycardia, hypotension, and abdominal pain. Irritability and mood swings, including depression and (rarely) mania, can occur. Clonidine may cause more sedation, dizziness, and hypotension than guanfacine. Rebound hypertension has occurred following abrupt discontinuation of either drug; gradual tapering is recommended.

Drug Interactions – Guanfacine is metabolized primarily by CYP3A4; dosage adjustments are recommended with concomitant use of strong or moderate CYP3A4 inhibitors or inducers.[31] Use with a tricyclic antidepressant could reduce the antihypertensive effect of an alpha$_2$-agonist. Concurrent administration of alpha$_2$-agonists and digoxin, calcium channel blockers, or beta blockers may result in additive cardiac effects such as bradycardia and AV block.

ATOMOXETINE — The selective norepinephrine reuptake inhibitor atomoxetine (*Strattera,* and generics) is FDA-approved for treatment of ADHD in both children and adults.[35] It is not a controlled substance. Atomoxetine was less effective than methylphenidate in reducing ADHD symptoms in a large randomized, double-blind clinical trial.[36] It has been used in patients who have not responded to or cannot tolerate stimulants and those for whom use of a controlled substance is unacceptable. Combination therapy with atomoxetine and a stimulant has been used off-label; limited evidence suggests that it may improve ADHD symptoms in some patients who have not responded adequately to stimulant monotherapy.[37]

Adverse Effects – The atomoxetine label contains a boxed warning about an increased risk of suicidal thoughts in children and adolescents. Somnolence, nausea, and vomiting have occurred in children starting atomoxetine, particularly when the initial dose is increased to the maximum dose within a few days. Atomoxetine has been associated with growth delays in the first 1-2 years of treatment; reductions in growth appear to be reversible in the long term.[38] Hepatitis has occurred rarely. Atomoxetine can cause small increases in blood pressure and heart rate in children.[25] It rarely can cause priapism; this effect appears to be more common with atomoxetine than with methylphenidate. As with stimulants, boys and men taking the drug should be instructed to seek medical attention immediately if priapism occurs.

Drug Interactions – Concurrent use of atomoxetine and an MAO inhibitor is contraindicated; atomoxetine should not be taken with or within 14 days after stopping an MAO inhibitor. Use of atomoxetine in patients who are CYP2D6 poor metabolizers or are taking strong CYP2D6 inhibitors[31] may result in increased atomoxetine serum concentrations; such patients can receive the recommended starting dose, but the dose should only be increased if it is well tolerated and symptoms fail to improve after 4 weeks of treatment.

PREGNANCY AND LACTATION

Use of **stimulants** during pregnancy has been increasing in recent years. A large cohort study of pregnant women in the US found a small increase in the risk of cardiac malformations with use of methylphenidate (relative risk [RR]: 1.27), but not with amphetamines, during the first trimester; the significance of this finding is unclear.[39,40] In another population-based cohort study, stimulant use during early pregnancy was associated with a small increased risk of preeclampsia (RR: 1.29). Late gestational exposure to stimulants resulted in an increase in the risk of preterm birth (RR: 1.30). **Atomoxetine** was not associated with any adverse outcomes, but the analyses may have been underpowered for this drug.[41,42] In animal studies, high doses of atomoxetine have resulted in adverse fetal effects. No adequate studies of **clonidine** or **guanfacine** in human pregnancy are available. In some animal studies with these drugs, fetal harm occurred with use of doses higher than the maximum recommended human dose.

Methylphenidate has been detected in human breast milk; there are no reports of adverse effects on the breastfed infant or of effects on milk production. Breastfeeding is not recommended during treatment with **amphetamines**. **Clonidine** is secreted in human breast milk. **Atomoxetine** and **guanfacine** have been found in the milk of lactating rats.

CHOICE OF DRUGS

Stimulants are the drugs of choice for treatment of ADHD symptoms. Factors to consider in choosing a stimulant formulation include onset and duration of action, ease of administration, and cost. Long-acting formulations are appropriate for most school-age children and adults.

A large meta-analysis of 133 randomized, double-blind trials compared the efficacy (based on outcomes reported after 12 weeks of treatment) and tolerability of various drugs used to treat ADHD in children and adults. When both efficacy and safety were considered, the authors concluded that the evidence supported use of methylphenidate for treatment of children and amphetamines for adults.[43]

Some expert clinicians have found that in clinical practice either stimulant class can be effective and well tolerated in both children and adults. Some patients may respond better to amphetamines than to methylphenidate and vice versa. The choice between them should be based on individual responses and preferences.

The FDA-approved **nonstimulants** appear to be less effective than stimulants in improving ADHD symptoms. They have been used to treat hyperactivity more than inattention. Nonstimulants can be used in combination with stimulants or when stimulants are contraindicated, ineffective, or not tolerated.[8]

A DEVICE

The FDA has authorized the marketing of an electrical nerve stimulation device *(Monarch eTNS [external Trigeminal Nerve Stimulation] System)* for children 7-12 years old with ADHD who are not currently taking a prescription ADHD drug. Evidence for the device's effectiveness is limited to one small (n=62) 5-week clinical trial in which nightly use reduced ADHD symptoms compared to sham treatment.[44]

1. HM Feldman and MI Reiff. Clinical practice. Attention deficit-hyperactivity disorder in children and adolescents. N Engl J Med 2014; 370:838.

2. ND Volkow and JM Swanson. Clinical practice: adult attention deficit-hyperactivity disorder. N Engl J Med 2013; 369:1935.

3. S Dalsgaard et al. Mortality in children, adolescents, and adults with attention deficit hyperactivity disorder: a nationwide cohort study. Lancet 2015; 385:2190.

4. SE McCabe et al. Age of onset, duration, and type of medication therapy for attention-deficit/hyperactivity disorder and substance use during adolescence: a multi-cohort national study. J Am Acad Child Adolesc Psychiatry 2016; 55:479.

5. Z Chang et al. Serious transport accidents in adults with attention-deficit/hyperactivity disorder and the effect of medication: a population-based study. JAMA Psychiatry 2014; 71:319.

6. P Lichtenstein et al. Medication for attention deficit-hyperactivity disorder and criminality. N Engl J Med 2012; 367:2006.

7. E Chan et al. Treatment of attention-deficit/hyperactivity disorder in adolescents: a systematic review. JAMA 2016; 315:1997.

8. ML Wolraich et al. Clinical practice guideline for the diagnosis, evaluation, and treatment of attention-deficit/hyperactivity disorder in children and adolescents. Pediatrics 2019; 144:e20192528.

9. D Coghill et al. Long-acting methylphenidate formulations in the treatment of attention-deficit/hyperactivity disorder: a systematic review of head-to-head studies. BMC Psychiatry 2013; 13:237.

10. QuilliChew ER – extended-release chewable methylphenidate tablets. Med Lett Drugs Ther 2016; 58:68.

11. Cotempla XR-ODT – another long-acting methylphenidate for ADHD. Med Lett Drugs Ther 2017; 59:183.

12. Quillivant XR – an extended-release oral suspension of methylphenidate. Med Lett Drugs Ther 2013; 55:10.

13. Transdermal methylphenidate (Daytrana) for ADHD. Med Lett Drugs Ther 2006; 48:49.

14. Jornay PM – evening-dosed methylphenidate for ADHD. Med Lett Drugs Ther 2019; 61:126.

15. Two new amphetamines for ADHD. Med Lett Drugs Ther 2016; 58:80.

16. A new amphetamine oral suspension (Adzenys ER) for ADHD. Med Lett Drugs Ther 2018; 60:e106.

17. RH Weisler et al. Efficacy and safety of SHP465 mixed amphetamine salts in the treatment of attention-deficit/hyperactivity disorder in adults: results of a randomized, double-blind, placebo-controlled, forced-dose clinical study. CNS Drugs 2017; 31:685.

18. M Brams et al. SHP465 mixed amphetamine salts in the treatment of attention-deficit/hyperactivity disorder in children and adolescents: results of a randomized, double-blind placebo-controlled study. J Child Adolesc Psychopharmacol 2018; 28:19.

19. Lisdexamfetamine dimesylate (Vyvanse) for ADHD. Med Lett Drugs Ther 2007; 49:58.

20. D Elbe et al. Focus on lisdexamfetamine: a review of its use in child and adolescent psychiatry. J Can Acad Child Adolesc Psychiatry 2010; 19:303.

21. JH Newcorn et al. Randomized, double-blind, placebo-controlled acute comparator trials of lisdexamfetamine and extended-release methylphenidate in adolescents with attention-deficit/hyperactivity disorder. CNS Drugs 2017; 31:999.

22. SC Cohen et al. Meta-analysis: risk of tics associated with psychostimulant use in randomized, placebo-controlled trials. J Am Acad Child Adolesc Psychiatry 2015; 54:728.

23. JM Swanson et al. Young adult outcomes in the follow-up of the multimodal treatment study of attention-deficit/hyperactivity disorder: symptom persistence, source discrepancy, and height suppression. J Child Psychol Psychiatry 2017; 58:663.

24. LV Moran et al. Psychosis with methylphenidate or amphetamine in patients with ADHD. N Engl J Med 2019; 380:1128.

25. L Hennissen et al. Cardiovascular effects of stimulant and non-stimulant medication for children and adolescents with ADHD: a systematic review and meta-analysis of trials of methylphenidate, amphetamines and atomoxetine. CNS Drugs 2017; 31:199.

26. WO Cooper et al. ADHD drugs and serious cardiovascular events in children and young adults. N Engl J Med 2011; 365:1896.

27. LA Habel et al. ADHD medications and risk of serious cardiovascular events in young and middle-aged adults. JAMA 2011; 306:2673.

28. H Schelleman et al. Cardiovascular events and death in children exposed and unexposed to ADHD agents. Pediatrics 2011; 127:1102.

29. SA Shahani et al. Attention deficit hyperactivity disorder screening electrocardiograms: a community-based perspective. Pediatr Cardiol 2014; 35:485.

30. LS Eiland et al. Priapism associated with the use of stimulant medications and atomoxetine for attention-deficit/hyperactivity disorder in children. Ann Pharmacother 2014; 48:1350.

31. Inhibitors and inducers of CYP enzymes and P-glycoprotein. Med Lett Drugs Ther 2019; November 6 (epub). Available at medicalletter.org/downloads/CYP_PGP_Tables.pdf.

32. ST Osland et al. Pharmacological treatment for attention deficit hyperactivity disorder (ADHD) in children with comorbid tic disorders. Cochrane Database Syst Rev 2018, 6:CD007990.

33. Guanfacine extended-release (Intuniv) for ADHD. Med Lett Drugs Ther 2010; 52:82.

34. Another extended-release alpha2-agonist for ADHD. Med Lett Drugs Ther 2011; 53:10.

35. Atomoxetine (Strattera) for ADHD. Med Lett Drugs Ther 2003; 45:11.

36. JH Newcorn et al. Atomoxetine and osmotically released methylphenidate for the treatment of attention deficit hyperactivity disorder: acute comparison and differential response. Am J Psychiatry 2008; 165:721.

37. T Treuer et al. A systematic review of combination therapy with stimulants and atomoxetine for attention-deficit/hyperactivity disorder, including patient characteristics, treatment strategies, effectiveness, and tolerability. J Child Adolesc Psychopharmacol 2013; 23:179.

38. VA Reed et al. The safety of atomoxetine for the treatment of children and adolescents with attention-deficit/hyperactivity disorder: a comprehensive review of over a decade of research. CNS Drugs 2016; 30:603.

39. KF Huybrechts et al. Association between methylphenidate and amphetamine use in pregnancy and risk of congenital malformations: a cohort study from the international pregnancy safety study consortium. JAMA Psychiatry 2018; 75:167.

40. C Andrade. Risk of major congenital malformations associated with the use of methylphenidate or amphetamines in pregnancy. J Clin Psychiatry 2018; 79(1):18f12108.

41. JM Cohen et al. Placental complications associated with psychostimulant use in pregnancy. Obstet Gynecol 2017; 130:1192.
42. C Andrade. Adverse gestational outcomes associated with attention-deficit/hyperactivity disorder medication exposure during pregnancy. J Clin Psychiatry 2018; 79(1):18f12136.
43. S Cortese et al. Comparative efficacy and tolerability of medications for attention-deficit hyperactivity disorder in children, adolescents, and adults: a systematic review and network meta-analysis. Lancet Psychiatry 2018; 5:727.
44. JJ McGough et al. Double-blind, sham-controlled, pilot study of trigeminal nerve stimulation for attention-deficit/hyperactivity disorder. J Am Acad Child Adolesc Psychiatry 2019; 58:403.

DRUGS FOR
Asthma

Original publication date – December 2020

The goal of asthma treatment is to control symptoms, prevent exacerbations, and maintain normal lung function.[1,2] Management of acute exacerbations of asthma in the emergency department is not discussed here.

ACUTE RELIEF OF SYMPTOMS

INHALED SABAs — The inhaled short-acting beta$_2$-agonists (SABAs) **albuterol** and **levalbuterol** are used for rapid relief of asthma symptoms. Their effect begins within 5 minutes, peaks within 15-60 minutes, and lasts for 4-6 hours. They do not decrease airway inflammation and should be used only as needed for relief of symptoms or for prevention of exercise-induced bronchoconstriction (EIB). In patients whose asthma is well controlled, SABAs should be needed infrequently (≤2 days/week). Racemic albuterol and levalbuterol are comparable to each other in safety and efficacy.

A new **epinephrine** hydrofluoroalkane (HFA) inhaler *(Primatene Mist)* is now available over the counter (OTC) for temporary relief of mild symptoms of intermittent asthma in patients ≥12 years old. It costs less than prescription inhalers, but use of inhaled epinephrine for self-treatment of asthma could result in delayed treatment of exacerbations and inadequate management of chronic asthma.

Adverse Effects – Inhaled SABAs can cause tremor, tachycardia, QT interval prolongation, hyperglycemia, hypokalemia, and hypomagnesemia, especially if used in high doses.

INHALED SAMA — The inhaled short-acting muscarinic antagonist (SAMA) **ipratropium bromide** is FDA-approved for treatment of chronic obstructive pulmonary disease (COPD), and has been used off-label for as-needed symptom relief in asthma patients who cannot tolerate a SABA and in combination with a SABA for treatment of acute bronchoconstriction. SABAs have a more rapid onset of action.

Adverse Effects – Ipratropium can cause dry mouth and pharyngeal irritation.

MAINTENANCE TREATMENT

INHALED CORTICOSTEROIDS — An inhaled corticosteroid (ICS) is the most effective maintenance treatment for asthma of any severity. In randomized, controlled trials, ICSs have been effective in preventing symptoms, exacerbations, and deaths due to asthma. At usual doses, all ICSs are similar in efficacy. Patients with well controlled asthma who stop using an ICS have an increased risk of exacerbations. In patients with mild asthma and poor adherence to regular ICS use, taking a low-dose ICS whenever a SABA is taken (off-label use) has been shown to reduce the risk of severe exacerbations.[3]

Adverse Effects – Local adverse effects of ICSs include oral candidiasis (thrush), dysphonia, and reflex cough and bronchospasm. Using a spacer (valved holding chamber) with a metered-dose inhaler and rinsing the mouth after inhalation may reduce these effects. Ciclesonide and beclomethasone dipropionate, prodrugs that are activated in the lungs, are less likely to cause oropharyngeal and systemic adverse effects.[4]

Regular use of low or medium doses of ICSs may reduce growth slightly, especially in prepubescent children. In one study, a medium dose of

---

Summary: Drugs for Asthma

▸ Inhaled short-acting beta₂-agonists (SABAs) can be used as needed for acute symptom relief and to prevent exercise-induced bronchoconstriction (EIB).

▸ An inhaled corticosteroid (ICS) is the most effective maintenance treatment for asthma of any severity.

▸ Daily treatment with a low dose of an ICS suppresses airway inflammation and reduces symptoms and exacerbations. As-needed use of a low-dose ICS plus a SABA or a low-dose ICS in combination with the long-acting beta₂-agonist (LABA) formoterol also reduces the risk of exacerbations.

▸ In patients who remain symptomatic despite adherence to ICS treatment and good inhalation technique, combination ICS/LABA plus as-needed SABA or ICS/formoterol single maintenance and reliever therapy (SMART) is recommended.

▸ In patients with asthma that is uncontrolled with medium- to high-dose ICS/LABA treatment, addition of an inhaled long-acting muscarinic antagonist (LAMA) improves lung function.

▸ In patients with moderate to severe allergic asthma, addition of the anti-IgE monoclonal antibody omalizumab has improved asthma control.

▸ In patients with moderate to severe eosinophilic asthma, addition of an anti-IL-5 monoclonal antibody (mepolizumab, reslizumab, or benralizumab) or the anti-IL-4 antibody dupilumab has reduced exacerbations and oral corticosteroid doses.

▸ In some patients with allergic asthma, allergen-specific immunotherapy may be helpful.

---

budesonide (400 mcg/day) for 4-6 years reduced mean adult height by 1.2 cm compared to placebo.[5]

Clinically relevant adverse effects on hypothalamic-pituitary-adrenal (HPA) axis function generally do not occur with low or medium doses of ICSs. Patients who require high-dose ICS treatment should be monitored for HPA axis suppression, changes in bone density, and development of cataracts or glaucoma.

INHALED LABAs — Addition of an inhaled long-acting beta₂-agonist (LABA) such as **salmeterol** or **formoterol** to an ICS improves lung function, decreases symptoms and exacerbations, and reduces rescue use of SABAs.

Table 1. Treatment of Asthma[1]

Asthma Severity	Recommended Regimen[2]
Mild intermittent	
Preferred	PRN SABA[3]
Alternatives	PRN low-dose ICS[4] + SABA PRN low-dose ICS[4]/formoterol[5]
Mild Persistent	
Preferred	Daily low-dose ICS[4] + PRN SABA PRN low-dose ICS[4] + SABA PRN low-dose ICS[4]/formoterol[5]
Alternatives	Daily leukotriene modifier or theophylline + PRN SABA
Moderate Persistent	
Preferred	Daily and PRN low- to medium-dose ICS[4]/formoterol[5]
Alternatives	Daily medium-dose ICS[4] + PRN SABA Daily low- to medium-dose ICS[4]/LABA + PRN SABA Daily low- to medium-dose ICS[4] + LAMA[6] or leukotriene modifier or theophylline + PRN SABA
Severe Persistent	
Preferred	Daily medium- to high-dose ICS[4]/LABA + LAMA[6] + PRN SABA[7]
Alternatives	Daily medium- to high-dose ICS[4]/LABA + PRN SABA[7] Daily high-dose ICS[4] + leukotriene modifier + PRN SABA[7] Daily high-dose ICS[4]/LABA + oral corticosteroid + PRN SABA[7]

ICS = inhaled corticosteroid; LABA = inhaled long-acting beta$_2$-agonist; LAMA = inhaled long-acting muscarinic antagonist; SABA = inhaled short-acting beta$_2$-agonist

1. Adapted from Expert Panel Working Group of the NHLBI. 2020 Focused Updates to the Asthma Management Guidelines. J Allergy Clin Immunol 2020; 146:1217 and the Global Initiative for Asthma. Global Strategy for Asthma Management and Prevention, 2020. (Available at: www.ginasthma.org. Accessed December 3, 2020).
2. For patients ≥12 years old. Treatment should be adjusted based on response.
3. As-needed SABA alone is no longer recommended by the Global Initiative for Asthma (GINA) for treatment of asthma in adolescents and adults because of an increased risk of severe exacerbations compared to regular or as-needed treatment with an ICS-containing regimen.
4. The ideal dose of an ICS is the lowest dose that maintains asthma control. Recommended low, medium, and high doses can be found at medicalletter.org/TML-article-1613b.
5. Data only available for low-dose budesonide/formoterol in a dry powder inhaler (not available in the US).
6. The LAMA tiotropium alone and the LAMA umeclidinium in combination with the ICS fluticasone and the LABA vilanterol in a single inhaler are FDA-approved for maintenance treatment of asthma.
7. If severe asthma remains uncontrolled, omalizumab can be added in patients with allergic asthma and an anti-interleukin (IL)-5 or anti-IL-4 antibody can be added in those with eosinophilic asthma. When other therapies fail, bronchial thermoplasty could be considered.

A low-dose ICS/formoterol combination can be used on an as-needed basis (off-label) instead of daily maintenance therapy with an ICS alone. The onset of action of formoterol is comparable to that of albuterol and is faster than that of salmeterol. Four randomized, 52-week trials in a total of >9500 patients ≥12 years old evaluated the efficacy of **as-needed budesonide/ formoterol** (in a dry powder inhaler; not available in the US) for treatment of mild or moderate asthma. As-needed budesonide/formoterol was at least as effective as budesonide maintenance therapy plus as-needed SABA for prevention of severe exacerbations, but it was less effective for asthma symptom control. Corticosteroid exposure was substantially reduced with as-needed therapy versus maintenance therapy.[6-9]

A meta-analysis of randomized trials that included >22,000 patients with persistent asthma found that using **budesonide/formoterol as single maintenance and reliever therapy (SMART)** reduced the risk of asthma exacerbations compared to using an ICS with or without a LABA as maintenance therapy and a SABA as reliever therapy.[10]

Adverse Effects – LABAs can cause tremor, hyperglycemia, hypokalemia, tachycardia, QT interval prolongation, and other cardiac effects. LABA monotherapy increases the risk of asthma-related death and is contra-indicated. A boxed warning about an increased risk of asthma-related hospitalization and death was removed from the labels of ICS/LABA combi-nation products in December 2017 because FDA-mandated safety trials comparing an ICS/LABA to an ICS alone in >41,000 adults and children with persistent asthma found that use of the combination was not associated with an increased risk of serious asthma-related adverse events.[11-13]

INHALED LAMAs — Tiotropium bromide, an inhaled long-acting muscarinic antagonist (LAMA), is FDA-approved for maintenance treat-ment of asthma in patients ≥6 years old. In patients with moderate to severe asthma, adding tiotropium to an ICS improves lung function and modestly decreases symptoms and the risk of exacerbations. In one study, use of an ICS plus a LAMA increased the risk of asthma-related hospital-ization and death in black patients, compared to ICS/LABA treatment.[1,14]

Table 2. Inhaled Short-Acting Bronchodilators for Asthma

Drug	Some Available Formulations
Inhaled Short-Acting Beta₂-Agonists (SABAs)	
Albuterol − *ProAir HFA* (Teva) generic *Proventil HFA* (Merck) generic *Ventolin HFA* (GSK) generic (Prasco)	HFA MDI (60² or 200 inh/unit) 90 mcg/inh
ProAir Respiclick (Teva)	DPI (200 inh/unit) 90 mcg/inh
*ProAir Digihaler*⁴ (Teva)	DPI (200 inh/unit) 90 mcg/inh
generic − single-dose vials	Solution for nebulization⁵ 0.63, 1.25, 2.5 mg/3 mL
Levalbuterol − *Xopenex HFA* (Sunovion)	HFA MDI (200 inh/unit) 45 mcg/inh
Xopenex (Sunovion) generic − single-dose vials	Solution for nebulization⁵ 0.31, 0.63, 1.25 mg/3 mL
Inhaled Epinephrine	
Primatene Mist (Amphastar)⁸	HFA MDI (160 inh/unit) 0.125 mg/inh
Inhaled Short-Acting Muscarinic Antagonist (SAMA)	
Ipratropium¹⁰ − *Atrovent HFA* (Boehringer Ingelheim)	HFA MDI (200 inh/unit) 17 mcg/inh
generic − single-dose vials	Solution for nebulization 500 mcg/2.5 mL
Inhaled Short-Acting Beta₂-Agonist/Short-Acting Muscarinic Antagonist Combination	
Albuterol/ipratropium¹⁰ − *Combivent Respimat* (Boehringer Ingelheim)	ISI (60, 120 inh/unit) 100 mcg/20 mcg/inh
generic	Solution for nebulization 2.5 mg/0.5 mg/3 mL

DPI = dry powder inhaler; HFA = hydrofluoroalkane; inh = inhalation; ISI = inhalation spray (soft mist) inhaler; MDI = metered-dose inhaler
1. Approximate WAC for 30 days' treatment at the lowest recommended adult dosage. WAC = wholesaler acquisition cost or manufacturer's published price to wholesalers; WAC represents a published catalogue or list price and may not represent an actual transactional price. Source: AnalySource® Monthly. November 5, 2020. Reprinted with permission by First Databank, Inc. All rights reserved. ©2020. www.fdbhealth.com/policies/drug-pricing-policy.
2. Only *Ventolin HFA* is available in a 60 inh/unit formulation.
3. Cost of 200 inhalations.
4. Contains a QR code and a built-in electronic module that automatically detects, records, and stores data on inhaler events such as date and time of inhalation and peak inspiratory flow rate. The device can pair with and transmit data to a mobile app via Bluetooth. The *ProAir Digihaler* contains a lithium-manganese dioxide battery.

Usual Adult Dosage	Usual Pediatric Dosage	Cost[1]
90-180 mcg q4-6h PRN	≥4 yrs: 90-180 mcg q4-6h PRN	$66.90[3]
		36.00[3]
		79.70[3]
		46.90[3]
		55.40[3]
		36.00[3]
90-180 mcg q4-6h PRN	≥4 yrs: 90-180 mcg q4-6h PRN	62.50[3]
90-180 mcg q4-6h PRN	≥4 yrs: 90-180 mcg q4-6h PRN	146.70[3]
1.25-5 mg q4-8h PRN	2-4 yrs: 0.63-2.5 mg q4-6h PRN	17.50[6]
90 mcg q4-6h PRN	≥4 yrs: 90 mcg q4-6h PRN	68.20[3]
0.63-1.25 mg tid q6-8h PRN	6-11 yrs: 0.31-0.63 mg tid q6-8h PRN	1044.00[7]
		170.00[7]
0.125-0.25 mg q4h PRN (max 1 mg/24 hrs)	≥12 yrs: 0.125-0.25 mg q4h PRN (max 1 mg/24 hrs)	28.00[9]
2 inh (34 mcg) qid PRN	––	411.40[3]
500 mcg qid PRN	––	15.00[7]
1 inh qid PRN	––	426.50[11]
2.5 mg/0.5 mg qid PRN	––	78.00[11]

5. Nebulized solutions may be used for very young, very old, and other patients unable to use pressurized aerosols. More time is required to administer the drug and the device may not be portable. Albuterol inhalation solution 0.5% is now available as a large-volume (20 mL) preservative-free concentrate (Med Lett Drugs Ther 2020; 62:173).
6. Cost of 100 2.5-mg doses.
7. Cost of 100 doses.
8. Available over the counter.
9. Approximate cost at www.walgreens.com. Accessed December 3, 2020.
10. Not FDA-approved for use in asthma.
11. Cost of 120 doses.

Addition of tiotropium to ICS/LABA treatment can improve lung function in patients with poorly controlled severe asthma and reduce the need for rescue oral corticosteroids, but it does not appear to lower the risk of exacerbations or improve symptoms.[14,15]

Other inhaled LAMAs are also effective for treatment of asthma. The three-drug inhaler containing the ICS fluticasone furoate, the LAMA **umeclidinium**, and the LABA vilanterol *(Trelegy Ellipta)*, previously approved for use in COPD, is now also FDA-approved for maintenance treatment of asthma in adults. In a randomized, double-blind trial in 2436 adults with uncontrolled moderate to severe asthma, the 3-drug combination improved lung function, but did not significantly reduce annualized asthma exacerbation rates, compared to fluticasone furoate/vilanterol.[16]

Adverse Effects – LAMAs have limited systemic absorption and are generally well tolerated. They commonly cause dry mouth. Pharyngeal irritation, increases in intraocular pressure, and urinary retention can occur.

LEUKOTRIENE MODIFIERS — The leukotriene receptor antagonists (LTRAs) **montelukast** and **zafirlukast** are alternatives to a low-dose ICS for patients who are unable or unwilling to use an ICS. Leukotriene modifiers are less effective than ICSs for asthma control. They are also generally less effective than inhaled LABAs as add-on therapy in patients whose asthma is not well controlled on an ICS alone. The 5-lipooxygenase inhibitor **zileuton** causes more adverse effects than LTRAs and is generally reserved for use as add-on therapy in severe asthma.

Adverse Effects – Neuropsychiatric events have occurred in patients taking leukotriene modifiers. The FDA now requires a boxed warning in the labeling of montelukast because serious neuropsychiatric events, including completed suicides, have been reported during and after its use.[17] Both zafirlukast and (especially) zileuton can cause life-threatening hepatic injury. Eosinophilic granulomatosis with polyangiitis (EGPA) has been reported rarely with montelukast and zafirlukast; in some cases, this was associated with withdrawal of oral corticosteroids.

THEOPHYLLINE — The availability of safer alternatives has significantly reduced the use of theophylline for persistent asthma. It is occasionally used in patients whose asthma is not controlled with an ICS and a LABA. Monitoring serum theophylline concentrations is recommended to maintain peak levels between 10 and 15 mcg/mL.

Adverse Effects – Theophylline can cause nausea, vomiting, nervousness, headache, and insomnia, and it interacts with many other drugs. At high serum concentrations, hypokalemia, hyperglycemia, tachycardia, cardiac arrhythmias, neuromuscular irritability, seizures, and death can occur.

ORAL CORTICOSTEROIDS — Oral corticosteroids are commonly used to treat severe exacerbations of asthma. They should be used as long-term controller medications only in the small minority of patients with poorly controlled severe persistent asthma.

FAILURE OF STANDARD TREATMENT — Failure of pharmacologic treatment often results from lack of adherence to prescribed medications, improper inhalation technique, uncontrolled comorbid conditions, misdiagnosis, or continued exposure to environmental irritants. Smoking and exposure to secondhand smoke can cause airway hyperresponsiveness and decrease the effectiveness of ICSs. Some patients with asthma who take aspirin or other NSAIDs may experience acute asthma symptoms. Oral or ophthalmic nonselective beta-adrenergic blockers, such as propranolol or timolol, can decrease the bronchodilating effect of both endogenous and exogenous beta$_2$-agonists in patients with asthma.

BIOLOGIC AGENTS — **Omalizumab** – Omalizumab *(Xolair),* a subcutaneously administered recombinant anti-IgE monoclonal antibody, is FDA-approved for use in patients ≥6 years old with moderate to severe persistent allergic asthma not well controlled on an ICS who have well-documented specific sensitizations to airborne allergens, such as mold, pollen, or animal dander. Addition of omalizumab to standard treatment has improved lung function and asthma control and decreased

Table 3. Inhaled Corticosteroids and Long-Acting Bronchodilators for Asthma

Drug	Some Available Formulations
Inhaled Corticosteroids (ICSs)[2]	
Beclomethasone dipropionate – QVAR Redihaler (Teva)	HFA MDI (120 inh/unit) 40, 80 mcg/inh
Budesonide – Pulmicort Flexhaler (AstraZeneca)	DPI (60, 120 inh/unit) 90, 180 mcg/inh
Pulmicort Respules (AstraZeneca) single-dose ampules generic	Suspension for nebulization[4] 0.25, 0.5 mg, 1 mg/2 mL
Ciclesonide – Alvesco (Sunovion)	HFA MDI (60 inh/unit) 80, 160 mcg/inh
Fluticasone furoate – Arnuity Ellipta (GSK)	DPI (14, 30 inh/unit) 50, 100, 200 mcg/inh
Fluticasone propionate – Flovent Diskus (GSK)	DPI (28, 60 inh/unit) 50, 100, 250 mcg/blister
Flovent HFA (GSK)	HFA MDI (120 inh/unit) 44, 110, 220 mcg/inh
ArmonAir Digihaler[6] (Teva)	DPI (60 inh/unit) 55, 113, 232 mcg/inh
Mometasone furoate – Asmanex HFA (Merck)	HFA MDI (120 inh/unit) 50, 100, 200 mcg/inh
Asmanex Twisthaler (Merck)	DPI (7, 30 inh/unit) 110 mcg/inh DPI (14, 30, 60, 120 inh/unit) 220 mcg/inh

DPI = dry powder inhaler; HFA = hydrofluoroalkane; inh = inhalation; ISI = inhalation spray (soft mist) inhaler; MDI = metered-dose inhaler
1. Approximate WAC for 30 days' treatment at the lowest recommended adult dosage. WAC = wholesaler acquisition cost or manufacturer's published price to wholesalers; WAC represents a published catalogue or list price and may not represent an actual transactional price. Source: AnalySource® Monthly. November 5, 2020. Reprinted with permission by First Databank, Inc. All rights reserved. ©2020. www.fdbhealth.com/policies/drug-pricing-policy.

Usual Adult Dosage	Usual Pediatric Dosage	Cost[1]
40-320 mcg bid[3]	4-11 yrs: 40-80 mcg bid	$190.20
180-720 mcg bid	6-17 yrs: 180-360 mcg bid	248.20
––	1-8 yrs: 0.25 mg bid or 0.5 mg once/day or bid or 1 mg once/day[3]	872.00[5] 238.00[5]
80-320 mcg bid[3]	≥12 yrs: 80-320 mcg bid[3]	274.20
100-200 mcg once/day[3]	5-11 yrs: 50 mcg once/day	178.80
100-1000 mcg bid[3]	4-11 yrs: 50-100 mcg bid[3]	192.80
88-880 mcg bid[3]	4-11 yrs: 88 mcg bid	192.80
55-232 mcg bid[3]	≥12 yrs: 55-232 mcg bid[3]	239.00
200-400 mcg bid[3]	5-11 yrs: 100-200 mcg bid[3]	191.40
220-440 mcg once/day in evening or 440 mcg bid[3]	4-11 yrs: 110 mcg once/day in evening[3]	191.60

2. Recommended low, medium, and high ICS doses can be found at medicalletter.org/TML-article-1613b.
3. Dose is based on disease severity and/or prior asthma therapy. See package insert.
4. May be used for very young, very old, and other patients unable to use pressurized aerosols.
5. Cost of 100 0.25-mg doses.
6. Contains a QR code and a built-in electronic module that automatically detects, records, and stores data on inhaler events such as date and time of inhalation and peak inspiratory flow rate. The device can pair with and transmit data to a mobile app via Bluetooth.

Continued on next page

Table 3. Inhaled Corticosteroids and Long-Acting Bronchodilators for Asthma (continued)

Drug	Some Available Formulations
Inhaled Long-Acting Beta$_2$-Agonists (LABAs)[7]	
Formoterol − *Perforomist* (Mylan)	Solution for nebulization[6] 20 mcg/2 mL
Salmeterol − *Serevent Diskus* (GSK)	DPI (28, 60 inh/unit) 50 mcg/blister
Inhaled Corticosteroid/Long-Acting Beta$_2$-Agonist Combinations	
Budesonide/formoterol − *Symbicort* (AstraZeneca)	HFA MDI (60, 120 inh/unit) 80, 160 mcg/4.5 mcg/inh
Fluticasone furoate/vilanterol − *Breo Ellipta* (GSK)	DPI (14, 30 inh/unit) 100, 200 mcg/25 mcg/inh

Fluticasone propionate/salmeterol −
   Advair Diskus (GSK)
   generic (Prasco)
   Wixela Inhub[9] (Mylan)
   Advair HFA (GSK)
 	
   AirDuo Respiclick (Teva)
   generic
   AirDuo Digihaler[6] (Teva)
	DPI (28, 60 inh/unit)[9]
	 100, 250, 500 mcg/50 mcg/blister
	
	 HFA MDI (60, 120 inh/unit)
	 45, 115, 230 mcg/ 21 mcg/inh
	 DPI (60 inh/unit)
	 55, 113, 232 mcg/14 mcg/inh
	 DPI (60 inh/unit)
	 55, 113, 232 mcg/14 mcg/inh

Mometasone/formoterol − *Dulera* (Merck)	HFA MDI (60, 120 inh/unit) 50, 100, 200 mcg/5 mcg/inh
Inhaled Long-Acting Muscarinic Antagonist (LAMA)	
Tiotropium − *Spiriva Respimat* (Boehringer Ingelheim)	ISI (60 inh/unit) 1.25 mcg/inh
Inhaled Corticosteroid/Long-Acting Muscarinic Antagonist/Long-Acting Beta$_2$-Agonist Combination	
Fluticasone furoate/umeclidinium/ vilanterol − *Trelegy Ellipta* (GSK)	DPI (14, 30 inh/unit) 100, 200 mcg/62.5 mcg/25 mcg/inh

DPI = dry powder inhaler; HFA = hydrofluoroalkane; inh = inhalation; ISI = inhalation spray (soft mist) inhaler; MDI = metered-dose inhaler
7. Only FDA-approved for concomitant use with an ICS in patients with asthma. Use as monotherapy is contraindicated.
8. Guidelines also recommend using ICS/formoterol as both maintenance and reliever therapy (Evidence only with budesonide/formoterol in a DPI; not an FDA-approved indication). Dosage for maintenance is 1-2 inh once/day or bid and for PRN use is 1-2 inh (max 12 inh/day [≥12 yrs] or 8 inh/day [4-11 yrs]) (see reference 1).

Usual Adult Dosage	Usual Pediatric Dosage	Cost[1]
20 mcg bid	——	1062.00
50 mcg bid	≥4 yrs: 50 mcg bid	399.20
2 inh bid[3,8]	6-11 yrs: 2 inh (80/4.5 mcg) bid[8]	$318.80
1 inh once/day[3]		361.80
1 inh bid[3]	4-11 yrs: 1 inh (100/50 mcg) bid	317.10 285.00 93.70
2 inh bid[3]	≥12 yrs: 2 inh bid[3]	317.10
1 inh bid[3]	≥12 yrs: 1 inh bid[3]	320.20 95.40
1 inh bid[3]	≥12 yrs: 1 inh bid[3]	399.00
2 inh (100 or 200 mcg/5 mcg) bid[3,8]	5-11 yrs: 2 inh (50 mcg/5 mcg) bid[8]	311.40
2 inh once/day	≥6 yrs: 2 inh once/day	455.20
1 inh once/day[3]	——	573.20

9. Generic equivalent of *Advair Diskus* that uses a different device. *Wixela Inhub* is only available in a 60 inh/unit formulation.

exacerbations, maintenance ICS doses, and hospitalizations in patients with allergic asthma, regardless of baseline eosinophil levels; improvements have been maintained for ≥4 years with continued treatment.[18]

Adverse Effects – Omalizumab can cause injection-site pain and bruising. Its labeling includes a boxed warning about a risk of anaphylaxis. Omalizumab should generally be administered in a healthcare setting by providers prepared to manage potentially life-threatening anaphylaxis. Self-administration at home in selected patients is under review by the FDA and is temporarily available during the COVID-19 pandemic. Symptoms of anaphylaxis can occur more than 2 hours post-injection. Patients receiving omalizumab should be advised to self-inject epinephrine promptly if anaphylaxis occurs.

Anti-Interleukin-5 (IL-5) Antibodies — The anti-IL-5 monoclonal antibodies mepolizumab *(Nucala)* and reslizumab *(Cinqair)* and the anti-IL-5 receptor alpha monoclonal antibody benralizumab *(Fasenra)* are FDA-approved for add-on maintenance treatment of severe eosinophilic asthma. SC injections of mepolizumab and benralizumab can be given at home with an autoinjector; reslizumab is administered by IV infusion over 20-50 minutes.

In patients with severe eosinophilic asthma, **mepolizumab** has reduced the frequency of clinically significant exacerbations by 40-60% compared to placebo; it has also had an oral corticosteroid-sparing effect (median dose reduced by 50% vs 0% with placebo).[19] In an open-label study in patients with uncontrolled severe eosinophilic asthma despite treatment with a high-dose ICS, other asthma controllers, and omalizumab, switching from omalizumab to mepolizumab significantly improved asthma control and reduced exacerbation rates.[20]

In patients with moderate to severe eosinophilic asthma, **reslizumab** reduced the frequency of clinically significant exacerbations by 54% compared to placebo.[21] It was more effective in patients with late-onset asthma (>40 years old) than in those with early-onset disease.[22] Reslizumab is not FDA-approved for use in patients <18 years old because the annual exacerbation rate in these patients was twice as high with the drug as with placebo.

Benralizumab has reduced exacerbation rates by about 30-50% in patients 12-75 years old with severe, uncontrolled eosinophilic asthma. In adults with severe eosinophilic asthma who had been taking oral corticosteroids for at least 6 months, addition of benralizumab significantly reduced median daily oral corticosteroid doses (by 75% vs 25% with placebo).[23]

Adverse Effects – The most common adverse effects of mepolizumab have been injection-site reactions, headache, back pain, and fatigue. Reslizumab has been associated with oropharyngeal pain, creatine phosphokinase elevations, myalgia, and, rarely, malignancies. Adverse effects that occurred more often with benralizumab than with placebo in clinical trials included headache, pyrexia, and pharyngitis. Hypersensitivity reactions have occurred with all three drugs; only reslizumab has a boxed warning in its labeling about a risk of anaphylaxis.

Anti-Interleukin-4 (IL-4) Antibody – **Dupilumab** *(Dupixent)*, an IL-4 receptor alpha subunit antagonist that inhibits IL-4 and IL-13 signaling, is FDA-approved for add-on maintenance treatment of moderate to severe asthma with an eosinophilic phenotype or oral corticosteroid-dependent asthma.[24] In 2 randomized, double-blind trials in >2700 patients receiving medium to high doses of inhaled corticosteroids plus 1 or 2 other asthma-controller medications, addition of dupilumab significantly decreased the annual rate of severe exacerbations by ~50-70% compared to placebo.[25,26] In a randomized, 24-week trial in 210 patients with severe asthma who were being treated with daily oral corticosteroids, addition of dupilumab resulted in a mean reduction in the oral corticosteroid dose of 70% versus 42% with addition of placebo.[27] Reductions in exacerbation rates and improvements in lung function have been sustained for up to 3 years with continued treatment.[28]

Table 4. Some Other Drugs for Asthma

Drug	Some Available Formulations
Leukotriene Modifiers	
Montelukast – generic *Singulair* (Merck)	10 mg tabs; 4, 5 mg chew tabs; 4 mg oral granules
Zafirlukast – generic *Accolate* (Par)	10, 20 mg tabs
Zileuton – *Zyflo* (Chiesi) extended-release – generic	600 mg tabs 600 mg ER tabs
Anti-Immunoglobulin E (IgE) Antibody	
Omalizumab – *Xolair* (Genentech)	150 mg single-dose vials; 75 mg/0.5 mL, 150 mg/mL single-dose prefilled syringes
Anti-Interleukin-5 (IL-5) and Anti-IL-5 Receptor Alpha Antibodies[7]	
Benralizumab – *Fasenra* (AstraZeneca)	30 mg/mL single-dose prefilled syringes, autoinjectors
Mepolizumab – *Nucala* (GSK)	100 mg single-dose vials; 100 mg/mL single- dose prefilled syringes, autoinjectors[8]
Reslizumab – *Cinqair* (Teva)	100 mg/10 mL single-use vials
Anti-Interleukin-4 (IL-4) Receptor Alpha Antibody	
Dupilumab – *Dupixent* (Sanofi/Regeneron)	200 mg/1.14 mL, 300 mg/2 mL single-dose prefilled syringes; 300 mL/2 mL single-dose prefilled pens

ER = extended-release
1. Approximate WAC for 30 days' treatment at the lowest recommended adult dosage. WAC = wholesaler acquisition cost or manufacturer's published price to wholesalers; WAC represents a published catalogue or list price and may not represent an actual transactional price. Source: AnalySource® Monthly. November 5, 2020. Reprinted with permission by First Databank, Inc. All rights reserved. ©2020. www.fdbhealth.com/policies/drug-pricing-policy.
2. Montelukast is taken once daily in the evening, with or without food. Montelukast granules must be taken within 15 minutes of opening the packet. Zafirlukast is taken 1 hour before or 2 hours after a meal. Zileuton is taken within one hour after morning and evening meals.
3. For exercise-induced bronchoconstriction (EIB), dose is one 10-mg tab for patients ≥15 years old and one 5-mg chewable tab for children 6-14 years old, taken at least 2 hours before exercise.
4. Dose for 12-23 months: one packet of 4-mg oral granules; 2-5 yrs: 4-mg chew tab or one packet of 4-mg oral granules; 6-14 yrs: 5-mg chew tab.

Usual Adult Dosage	Usual Pediatric Dosage	Cost[1]
10 mg PO once/day in evening[2,3]	≥1 yr: 4 or 5 mg PO once/day in evening[2-4]	$9.90 228.30
20 mg PO bid[2]	5-11 yrs: 10 mg PO bid[2] ≥12 yrs: 20 mg PO bid[2]	91.00 227.60
600 mg PO qid[2]	≥12 yrs: 600 mg PO qid[2]	3759.00
1200 mg PO bid[2]	≥12 yrs: 1200 mg PO bid[2]	3222.00
150-300 mg SC q4 wks or 225-375 mg SC q2 wks[5]	6-11 yrs: 75-300 mg SC q4 wks or 225-375 mg q2 wks[5]	1128.50[6]
30 mg SC q4 wks x 3, then q8 wks	≥12 yrs: 30 mg SC q4 wks x 3, then q8 wks	5043.70[6]
100 mg SC q4 wks	6-11 yrs: 40 mg SC q4 wks ≥12 yrs: 100 mg SC q4 wks	3074.10[6]
3 mg/kg IV q4 wks	––	2853.00[6]
400 mg SC then 200 mg q2 wks or 600 mg SC then 300 mg q2 wks[9,10]	≥12 yrs: 400 mg SC then 200 mg q2 wks or 600 mg SC then 300 mg q2 wks[9,10]	3110.10[11]

5. Dose depends on the patient's body weight and total serum IgE level. See package insert for specific dosing instructions.
6. Cost of a single treatment. With reslizumab, cost is for a patient weighing 70 kg (3 vials).
7. Mepolizumab and reslizumab target IL-5 itself and benralizumab targets the IL-5 receptor alpha subunit.
8. Prefilled syringes and autoinjectors are only for use in patients ≥12 years old.
9. The initial loading dose is administered as 2 injections at different sites.
10. The dose for patients with oral corticosteroid-dependent asthma or comorbid moderate to severe atopic dermatitis is 600 mg SC then 300 mg every 2 weeks.
11. Cost of two 200-mg doses.

Continued on next page

Table 4. Some Other Drugs for Asthma (continued)	
Drug	Some Available Formulations
Theophylline[12]	
generic	100, 200, 300, 400, 450, 600 mg ER tabs; 80 mg/15 mL soln
Elixophyllin (Nostrum Labs)	80 mg/15 mL soln
Theo-24 (Auxilium)	100, 200, 300, 400 mg ER caps

ER = extended-release
12. Extended-release formulations may not be interchangeable.
13. If *Theo-24* is taken <1 hr before a high-fat content meal, the entire 24-hour dose can be released in a 4-hour period.

Adverse Effects – In clinical trials, the most common adverse effect of dupilumab was injection-site reactions (14-18%). Eosinophilic pneumonia and vasculitis consistent with EGPA have been reported; a causal relationship has not been established. Conjunctivitis has occurred in patients treated with dupilumab. Transient increases in blood eosinophils are common. Anaphylaxis has occurred rarely.

ALLERGEN IMMUNOTHERAPY — In some patients with allergic asthma, specific immunotherapy may produce long-lasting reductions in asthma symptoms, exacerbations, and the need for medications.[29] Currently available evidence favors the use of subcutaneous injections over sublingual tablets.[1]

BRONCHIAL THERMOPLASTY — Approved by the FDA for use in adults with severe persistent asthma not well controlled on an ICS and a LABA, bronchial thermoplasty does not improve lung function, but it does modestly improve asthma-specific quality of life, and it has reduced exacerbation rates; these effects have been reported to last for up to 5 years.[30] The long-term efficacy and safety of the procedure are unknown. Worsening of asthma, hemoptysis, atelectasis, and lower respiratory tract infections requiring hospitalization have occurred during and after treatment.[1,31]

Usual Adult Dosage	Usual Pediatric Dosage	Cost[1]
300-600 mg PO once/day or divided bid	12-20 mg/kg/day (max 600 mg/day)[14]	$15.80
300-600 mg/day PO divided tid-qid		1260.30
300-600 mg PO once/day[13]		82.20

14. Dosing for infants: 0.2 x (age in weeks) + 5 = dose in mg/kg/day. Recommended dosing interval varies with different formulations (see package inserts).

EXERCISE-INDUCED BRONCHOCONSTRICTION — Use of a SABA just before exercise prevents EIB for 2-4 hours after inhalation. In patients who continue to have symptoms despite use of a SABA before exercise or who require daily use of a SABA, ICS maintenance treatment should be started or its dosage increased. The leukotriene modifier montelukast is FDA-approved for prevention of EIB; it has been shown to be effective as soon as 2 hours and as long as 24 hours after administration.

PREGNANCY — Poorly controlled asthma symptoms and acute exacerbations increase the risk of complications, including pre-eclampsia, cesarean section, perinatal mortality, preterm birth, and low birth weight.[32]

Albuterol is the preferred SABA for use in pregnancy. **ICSs (budesonide** is the best studied) are preferred for maintenance treatment during pregnancy; they reduce the risk of exacerbations in the mother and do not appear to adversely affect fetal adrenal function. **LABAs** (used with ICSs), **theophylline**, and **montelukast** appear to be safe for use during pregnancy. Teratogenicity in animals has been reported with **zileuton**.

A prospective observational study in 230 pregnant women exposed to **omalizumab**, 83% of whom were exposed during all 3 trimesters of their pregnancy, found no evidence of an increased risk of major congenital anomalies.[33] **Allergen immunotherapy** and omalizumab should gener-ally not be initiated during pregnancy, but they can be continued (without dose escalation) in patients already receiving them. No adequate studies of the **anti-IL-5 antibodies** in pregnant women are available; there was no evidence of fetal harm in animal studies. Case reports of **dupilumab** use in pregnant women have not shown a drug-associated risk of adverse maternal or fetal outcomes, but more data are needed.

1. Expert Panel Working Group of the NHLBI. 2020 focused updates to the asthma management guidelines: a report from the National Asthma Education and Prevention Program Coordinating Committee Expert Panel Working Group. J Allergy Clin Immunol 2020; 146:1217.
2. Global Initiative for Asthma. Global strategy for asthma management and prevention (2020 update). Available at www.ginasthma.org. Accessed December 3, 2020.
3. K Sumino et al. A pragmatic trial of symptom-based inhaled corticosteroid use in African-American children with mild asthma. J Allergy Clin Immunol Pract 2020; 8:176.
4. JK Mukker et al. Ciclesonide: a pro-soft drug approach for mitigation of side effects of inhaled corticosteroids. J Pharm Sci 2016; 105:2509.
5. HW Kelly et al. Effect of inhaled glucocorticoids in childhood on adult height. N Engl J Med 2012; 367:904.
6. PM O'Byrne et al. Inhaled combined budesonide-formoterol as needed in mild asthma. N Engl J Med 2018; 378:1865.
7. ED Bateman et al. As-needed budesonide-formoterol versus maintenance budesonide in mild asthma. N Engl J Med 2018; 378:1877.
8. R Beasley et al. Controlled trial of budesonide-formoterol as needed for mild asthma. N Engl J Med 2019; 380:2020.
9. J Hardy et al. Budesonide-formoterol reliever therapy versus maintenance budesonide plus terbutaline reliever therapy in adults with mild to moderate asthma (PRACTICAL): a 52-week, open-label, multicentre, superiority, randomised controlled trial. Lancet 2019; 394:919.
10. DM Sobieraj et al. Association of inhaled corticosteroids and long-acting β-agonists as controller and quick relief therapy with exacerbations and symptom control in persistent asthma: a systematic review and meta-analysis. JAMA 2018; 319:1485.
11. DA Stempel et al. Safety of adding salmeterol to fluticasone propionate in children with asthma. N Engl J Med 2016; 375:840.
12. WW Busse et al. Combined analysis of asthma safety trials of long-acting β$_2$-agonists. N Engl J Med 2018; 378:2497.
13. FDA Drug Safety Communication. December 20, 2017. Available at: www.fda.gov/Drugs/DrugSafety/ucm589587.htm. Accessed December 3, 2020.
14. DM Sobieraj et al. Association of inhaled corticosteroids and long-acting muscarinic antagonists with asthma control in patients with uncontrolled, persistent asthma: a systematic review and meta-analysis. JAMA 2018; 319:1473.

15. KM Kew and K Dahri. Long-acting muscarinic antagonists (LAMA) added to combination long-acting beta2-agonists and inhaled corticosteroids (LABA/ICS) versus LABA/ICS for adults with asthma. Cochrane Database Syst Rev 2016; 1:CD011721.

16. LA Lee et al. Efficacy and safety of once-daily single-inhaler triple therapy (FF/UMEC/VI) versus FF/VI in patients with inadequately controlled asthma (CAPTAIN): a double-blind, randomised, phase 3A trial. Lancet Respir Med 2020 Sep 9 (epub).

17. In brief: Neuropsychiatric events with montelukast. Med Lett Drugs Ther 2020; 62:65.

18. KM MacDonald et al. Short- and long-term real-world effectiveness of omalizumab in severe allergic asthma: systematic review of 42 studies published 2008-2018. Expert Rev Clin Immunol 2019; 15:553.

19. Mepolizumab (Nucala) for severe eosinophilic asthma. Med Lett Drugs Ther 2016; 58:11.

20. KR Chapman et al. The clinical benefit of mepolizumab replacing omalizumab in uncontrolled severe eosinophilic asthma. Allergy 2019; 74:1716.

21. Reslizumab (Cinqair) for severe eosinophilic asthma. Med Lett Drugs Ther 2016; 58:81.

22. G Brusselle et al. Reslizumab in patients with inadequately controlled late-onset asthma and elevated blood eosinophils. Pulm Pharmacol Ther 2017; 43:39.

23. Benralizumab (Fasenra) for severe eosinophilic asthma. Med Lett Drugs Ther 2018; 60:33.

24. Dupilumab (Dupixent) for asthma. Med Lett Drugs Ther 2019; 61:6.

25. S Wenzel et al. Dupilumab efficacy and safety in adults with uncontrolled persistent asthma despite use of medium-to-high-dose inhaled corticosteroids plus a long-acting β_2 agonist: a randomised double-blind placebo-controlled pivotal phase 2b dose-ranging trial. Lancet 2016; 388:31.

26. M Castro et al. Dupilumab efficacy and safety in moderate-to-severe uncontrolled asthma. N Engl J Med 2018; 378:2486.

27. KF Rabe et al. Efficacy and safety of dupilumab in glucocorticoid-dependent severe asthma. N Engl J Med 2018; 378:2475.

28. M Wechsler et al. Dupilumab is well tolerated and shows sustained efficacy in patients with asthma: Liberty Asthma Traverse. 78th Annual Scientific Meeting of the American College of Allergy, Asthma & Immunology (ACAAI); virtual meeting; Nov. 13-15, 2020. Abstract P219.

29. K Xu et al. Efficacy of add-on sublingual immunotherapy for adults with asthma: a meta-analysis and systematic review. Ann Allergy Asthma Immunol 2018; 121:186.

30. NC Thomson. Recent developments in bronchial thermoplasty for severe asthma. J Asthma Allergy 2019; 12:375.

31. PI Bonta et al. Bronchial thermoplasty in severe asthma: best practice recommendations from an expert panel. Respiration 2018; 95:289.

32. H Wang et al. Asthma in pregnancy: pathophysiology, diagnosis, whole-course management, and medication safety. Can Respir J 2020; 2020:9046842.

33. JA Namazy et al. Pregnancy outcomes in the omalizumab pregnancy registry and a disease-matched comparator cohort. J Allergy Clin Immunol 2020; 145:528.

DRUGS FOR
Atopic Dermatitis

Original publication date − June 2020

Atopic dermatitis (AD; also known as eczema) is frequently associated with other atopic disorders such as allergic rhinitis, asthma, and food allergy. It commonly presents in infancy and early childhood and has a relapsing course, often improving by adolescence, but sometimes persisting into (or first appearing in) adulthood or even old age.[1,2]

NONPHARMACOLOGIC THERAPY

Skin hydration (a daily bath) followed immediately by application of an **emollient** is highly recommended. Emollients can improve signs and symptoms of AD and reduce the number of flares and the need for topical anti-inflammatory medication.[3] The results of a few small studies suggested that use of emollients could prevent AD in infants from high-risk families, but a randomized, controlled trial in 1394 newborns with a family history of AD, asthma, or allergic rhinitis found that daily emollient use during the first year was not more effective than standard skin care in preventing AD.[4]

TOPICAL THERAPY

CORTICOSTEROIDS — Topical corticosteroids are recommended for first-line treatment of AD when nonpharmacologic therapies have failed. Low-, medium-, and high-potency formulations are available (see Table 1).

Summary: Drugs for Atopic Dermatitis

- ► A daily bath followed by application of an emollient is recommended for all patients with atopic dermatitis.
- ► Topical corticosteroids are generally used to treat inflammation in atopic dermatitis. Once remission has been achieved, the least potent topical corticosteroid that is effective should be used for maintenance treatment.
- ► Topical calcineurin inhibitors do not cause skin atrophy and can be used on the face or intertriginous areas. They can also be used as maintenance treatment to minimize use of topical corticosteroids.
- ► Crisaborole ointment is a relatively new drug that was modestly effective in two 28-day clinical trials in patients with mild to moderate atopic dermatitis and is generally well tolerated.
- ► UV phototherapy can be used when topical therapies have failed. Narrowband UVB is generally recommended.
- ► The subcutaneously injected interleukin (IL)-4 and IL-13 antagonist dupilumab is effective in patients with moderate to severe disease that has not responded to topical therapies.
- ► Cyclosporine (used off-label) has been effective for treatment of moderate to severe disease. Its efficacy may be comparable to that of dupilumab, but cyclosporine has more adverse effects.
- ► Oral antihistamines have not been shown to be effective for treatment of atopic dermatitis.

A medium- or high-potency topical corticosteroid may be needed to achieve control of skin inflammation. High-potency corticosteroids such as betamethasone dipropionate 0.05% ointment or cream should only be applied to the trunk and extremities and never to the face or intertriginous areas such as the axillae and groin. Low-potency corticosteroids such as hydrocortisone cream are safe for use on the face and intertriginous areas. For treatment of active lesions, topical corticosteroids are applied twice daily. For maintenance treatment, the least potent topical corticosteroid that is effective should be used once or twice weekly.

Adverse Effects – Long-term use of topical corticosteroids can lead to development of skin atrophy, purpura, telangiectasias, and permanent striae. When applied to the eyelids for prolonged periods, they can cause glaucoma and cataracts. The risk of adrenal suppression is low;

it increases with corticosteroid potency, percentage of body surface covered, and duration of treatment.[5] The risk of adverse effects is greatest when high-potency corticosteroids are applied under occlusive dressings in infants and young children with widespread skin involvement who require long-term treatment. Adverse effects are rare with low- to medium-potency topical corticosteroids.[6]

Pregnancy and Lactation – Low- to medium-potency topical corticosteroids appear to be safe for use during pregnancy and lactation.

CALCINEURIN INHIBITORS — Topical tacrolimus (*Protopic,* and generics) and pimecrolimus (*Elidel,* and generics) are FDA-approved for second-line treatment of mild to moderate (pimecrolimus) or moderate to severe (tacrolimus) AD in patients ≥2 years old (tacrolimus 0.03% and pimecrolimus) or ≥ 16 years old (tacrolimus 0.1%). Calcineurin inhibitors are similar in efficacy to low- to medium-potency corticosteroids.[7] Applied twice daily, they can reduce inflammation and itching associated with AD within a few days.[8] They can be used on the face and intertriginous areas, where corticosteroid adverse effects can be troublesome. They can also be used as maintenance treatment to minimize use of topical corticosteroids. In patients whose disease had stabilized following acute treatment, application of topical tacrolimus 2-3 times weekly for up to 1 year increased the number of flare-free days and the time to relapse.[7]

Adverse Effects – Tacrolimus and, less often, pimecrolimus can cause mild, transient itching, burning, stinging, and erythema, but they do not cause cutaneous atrophy. Both drugs have been associated with an increased risk of viral skin infections such as herpes simplex and varicella zoster. The FDA has required a boxed warning in the labels of topical calcineurin inhibitors about rare cases of lymphoma and other cancers associated with prolonged treatment. A causal effect is difficult to establish because AD itself, particularly severe AD, has been associated with an increased risk of lymphoma. A large cohort study with a median follow-up of 2-6 years found that, compared to use of medium- or high-potency

Table 1. Some Topical Corticosteroids for Atopic Dermatitis

Drug	Vehicle	Cost[1]
Super-High Potency		
Betamethasone dipropionate 0.05% augmented		
generic	oint	$118.40/50 g
Diprolene (Merck)		202.50/50 g
Clobetasol propionate 0.05%		
generic	oint, cream, gel	34.70/30 g
	lotion, soln	121.90/59 mL
	foam	155.70/50 g
Temovate (Sandoz)	oint, cream	267.50/30 g
Clobex (Galderma)	spray	442.50/59 mL
Olux, Olux-E (Mylan)	foam	536.30/50 g
Fluocinonide 0.1%		
generic	cream	128.00/30 g
Vanos (Bausch)		952.30/30 g
Halobetasol propionate 0.05%		
generic	oint, cream	153.10/50 g
Ultravate (Ranbaxy)	lotion	916.00/50 g
High Potency		
Amcinonide 0.1%	oint	324.00/60 g
Betamethasone dipropionate 0.05% augmented	cream	17.40/30 g
Betamethasone dipropionate 0.05%	oint	98.40/45 g
Desoximethasone 0.25%		
generic	oint, cream	55.10/60 g
Topicort (Taro)	oint, cream, spray	343.60/60 g
Desoximethasone 0.05%	gel	276.00/60 g
Diflorasone diacetate 0.05%		
generic	oint	335.50/30 g
ApexiCon E (Sandoz)	cream	563.00/30 g

oint = ointment; soln = solution

1. Approximate WAC. WAC = wholesaler acquisition cost or manufacturer's published price to wholesalers; WAC = wholesaler acquisition cost or manufacturer's published price to wholesalers; WAC represents a published catalogue or list price and may not represent an actual transactional price. Source: Analy-Source® Monthly. May 5, 2020. Reprinted with permission by First Databank, Inc. All rights reserved. ©2020. www.fdbhealth.com/policies/drug-pricing-policy. When multiple formulations are listed, the price of the first formulation is provided.

Continued on next page

Table 1. Some Topical Corticosteroids for Atopic Dermatitis (continued)

Drug	Vehicle	Cost[1]
High Potency (continued)		
Fluocinonide 0.05%	oint, gel	$75.31/30 g
	cream, soln	72.90/30 g
Halcinonide 0.1%		
Halog (Sun)	oint, cream	770.10/60 g
Medium-High Potency		
Amcinonide 0.1%	cream	189.00/30 g
	lotion	271.40/60 mL
Betamethasone dipropionate 0.05%	cream	60.00/45 g
Betamethasone valerate 0.1%	oint	33.20/45 g
Betamethasone valerate 0.12%		
generic	foam	171.90/50 g
Luxiq (Prestium/Mylan)		447.80/50 g
Desoximethasone 0.05%	cream	293.50/60 g
Diflorasone diacetate 0.05%	cream	335.50/30 g
Fluocinonide emollient 0.05%	cream	55.10/30 g
Fluticasone propionate 0.005%	oint	22.30/30 g
Mometasone furoate 0.1%	oint	21.00/45 g
Triamcinolone acetonide 0.5%	oint, cream	14.00/30 g
Medium Potency		
Betamethasone dipropionate 0.05%		
Sernivo (Encore)	spray	902.95/120 mL
Clocortolone pivalate 0.1%		
generic	cream	268.70/45 g
Cloderm (Promius)		341.70/45 g
Fluocinolone acetonide 0.025%	oint	58.50/30 g
Flurandrenolide 0.05%		
generic	oint	564.10/60 g
Cordran (Aqua)		738.80/60 g
Hydrocortisone valerate 0.2%	oint	158.70/45 g
Mometasone furoate 0.1%	cream, soln	30.00/45 g
Triamcinolone acetonide 0.1%	oint, cream	8.30/30 g
Triamcinolone acetonide 0.05%	oint	779.30/430 g

oint = ointment; soln = solution

Continued on next page

Table 1. Some Topical Corticosteroids for Atopic Dermatitis (continued)		
Drug	**Vehicle**	**Cost[1]**
Medium-Low Potency		
Betamethasone dipropionate 0.05%	lotion	$32.80/60 mL
Betamethasone valerate 0.1%	cream	40.30/30 g
Desonide 0.05%	oint	45.00/30 g
Fluocinolone acetonide 0.025%	cream	58.50/30 g
Flurandrenolide 0.05%		
generic	cream, lotion	825.30/120 g
Cordran (Aqua)		1224.00/120 g
Fluticasone propionate 0.05%		
generic	cream	22.20/30 g
Cutivate (Sandoz)		113.10/30 g
Hydrocortisone butyrate 0.1%		
generic	cream, oint	62.50/45 g
	lotion, soln	386.00/59 mL
Locoid Lipocream (Bausch)	cream	62.50/45 g
Hydrocortisone probutate 0.1%		
Pandel (Sandoz)	cream	1072.70/80 g
Hydrocortisone valerate 0.2%	cream	63.00/45 g
Prednicarbate 0.1%	cream, oint	114.30/30 g
Triamcinolone acetonide 0.025%	oint	6.10/30 g
Triamcinolone acetonide 0.1%	lotion	23.90/60 mL
Low Potency		
Alclometasone dipropionate 0.05%	cream, oint	76.90/30 g
Betamethasone valerate 0.1%	lotion	60.00/60 mL
Desonide 0.05%		
generic	cream	49.50/30 g
	lotion	236.90/59 mL
Desonate (Bayer)	gel	631.00/60 g
Verdeso (Stiefel)	foam	992.40/100 g
Fluocinolone acetonide 0.01%	cream	74.20/30 g
	soln	33.60/60 mL
Triamcinolone acetonide 0.025%	cream	5.50/30 g
	lotion	29.00/60 mL
oint = ointment; soln = solution		

Continued on next page

Table 1. Some Topical Corticosteroids for Atopic Dermatitis (continued)		
Drug	**Vehicle**	**Cost[1]**
Lowest Potency		
Hydrocortisone 2.5%	cream, oint	$4.20/30 g
	lotion	30.00/59 mL
Hydrocortisone 1.0%[2]	oint	5.00/28 g[3]
	cream	3.80/28 g[3]
Hydrocortisone 0.5%[2]	cream	1.75/30 g
oint = ointment; soln = solution 2. Available without a prescription. 3. Price according to walgreens.com. Accessed June 4, 2020.		

topical corticosteroids, initiating treatment with topical tacrolimus was associated with an increased risk of lymphoma in children (incidence rate ratio [IRR] 3.74) and cutaneous T-cell lymphoma in adults (IRR 1.76); the IRR increased with higher cumulative doses of tacrolimus. The incidence rate per 100,000 person-years, however, was low in both children (10.4) and adults (9.5). The authors state that residual confounding by severity of atopic dermatitis, increased monitoring of severe patients, and reverse causation could have affected the results.[9]

Pregnancy and Lactation – Data on the use of topical tacrolimus and pimecrolimus in pregnant women are limited. In animals given oral tacrolimus, maternal and fetal toxicity occurred at doses equivalent to less than the maximum recommended human dose (MRHD). Use of oral tacrolimus in pregnant women has been associated with neonatal hyperkalemia and renal dysfunction. In dermal embryofetal development studies of pimecrolimus in animals, teratogenicity was not observed at doses equivalent to 0.65 times the MRHD; maternal and fetal toxicity occurred with very high oral doses of the drug.

Tacrolimus has been detected in human breast milk; it is not known whether pimecrolimus is excreted in human milk. Use of these drugs while breastfeeding is not recommended.

CRISABOROLE — Crisaborole *(Eucrisa)*, a topical phosphodies-terase type-4 (PDE4) inhibitor, is FDA-approved for treatment of mild to moderate AD in patients ≥3 months old.[10] It acts in part by increasing levels of cyclic adenosine monophosphate (cAMP), which suppresses production of proinflammatory cytokines in the skin. Systemic absorption is minimal.

In two randomized trials comparing crisaborole 2% ointment applied twice daily for 28 days to its vehicle alone in a total of 1522 patients ≥2 years old with mild to moderate AD, a statistically significantly higher percentage of patients using crisaborole achieved clear or almost-clear skin (33% vs 25% and 31% vs 18%).[11] How crisaborole compares to topical corticosteroids or calcineurin inhibitors for treatment of AD remains to be determined.[12]

Adverse Effects – The main adverse effects of crisaborole in clinical trials have been stinging and burning at the application site. Contact urticaria occurred in <1% of patients. In an open-label 48-week extension study in 517 patients ≥ 2 years old who had completed the 28-day vehicle-controlled trials, treatment-related adverse effects occurred in 10% of patients, were similar to those reported in the 28-day trials, and did not increase over time; only 2% of patients discontinued the drug because of adverse effects.[13] In an open-label 28-day study, crisaborole appeared to be safe for use in infants 3 to <24 months old with mild to moderate AD.[14]

Pregnancy and Lactation – There are no adequate studies of crisaborole in pregnant women. No adverse effects on embryofetal development were observed in pregnant rabbits and rats given oral crisaborole at doses up to 3 and 5 times, respectively, the MRHD. No information is available on the presence of the drug in human breast milk or on its effects on the breastfed infant or milk production.

COAL TAR — Coal tar preparations have antipruritic and anti-inflammatory effects, but they are messy and odoriferous and are seldom used now except in shampoo formulations. Adverse effects include skin irritation, folliculitis, and photosensitivity.

PHOTOTHERAPY

UV phototherapy has been effective in some patients with AD after failure of topical drugs. It can be used alone or in combination with emollients and topical corticosteroids.[15] Use with topical calcineurin inhibitors, cyclosporine, or azathioprine should be avoided because of a possible increase in the risk of skin cancer. Oral or topical psoralens combined with UVA radiation (PUVA) is effective, but can increase the risk of skin cancer. Narrowband UVB is safer and is the most frequently recommended phototherapy; a review of randomized trials found that it was more effective than other types of phototherapy for management of AD.[16] Phototherapy is usually administered 2-3 times per week and is discontinued if no improvement occurs within 4-8 weeks. It may not be available or practical for many patients.[17]

Adverse Effects – Itching, burning, stinging, dryness, erythema, tenderness, and altered pigmentation can occur.

Pregnancy and Lactation – Narrowband UVB is considered safe for use during pregnancy. Breastfeeding should be avoided for at least 24 hours after PUVA; UVB phototherapy is preferred for women who are breastfeeding.

SYSTEMIC THERAPY

Systemic drugs are recommended when AD is inadequately controlled with topical drugs and/or phototherapy.[18]

DUPILUMAB — Dupilumab *(Dupixent)* is a subcutaneously injected, fully human, IgG4 monoclonal antibody that binds to the interleukin (IL)-4 receptor alpha subunit shared by IL-4 and IL-13 receptors, inhibiting the signaling of these inflammatory cytokines. It is FDA-approved

Table 2. Topical Nonsteroidal and Some Systemic Drugs for Atopic Dermatitis

Drug	Some Available Formulations
Topical	
Calcineurin Inhibitors	
Pimecrolimus – generic *Elidel* (Bausch)	1% cream (30, 60, and 100 g tubes)
Tacrolimus – generic *Protopic* (Leo)	0.03%, 0.1% ointment (30, 60 and 100 g tubes)
PDE4 Inhibitor	
Crisaborole – *Eucrisa* (Pfizer)	2% ointment (60 and 100 g tubes)
Systemic	
IL-4/13 Antagonist	
Dupilumab – *Dupixent* (Sanofi/Regeneron)	200 mg/1.14 mL, 300 mg/2 mL single-dose prefilled syringes
Immunosuppressants	
Cyclosporine[5] – generic *Neoral* (Novartis) *Gengraf* (Abbvie)	25, 50, 100 mg caps; 100 mg/mL PO soln 25, 100 mg caps; 100 mg/mL PO soln
Methotrexate oral[5,7] – generic	2.5 mg tabs
injectable[5,7] – generic *Otrexup* (Antares) *Rasuvo* (Medac)	25 mg/mL single-dose vials 10, 12.5, 15, 17.5, 20, 22.5, 25 mg single-dose auto injectors 7.5, 10, 12.5, 15, 17.5, 20, 22.5, 25, 27.5, 30 mg single-dose auto-injectors
Azathioprine[5] – generic *Imuran* (Sebela) *Azasan* (Salix)	50 mg tabs 75, 100 mg tabs

soln = solution
1. Dosage adjustment may be needed for renal or hepatic impairment (immunosuppressants).
2. Approximate WAC for a 60-g tube (topical drugs) or for 3 months' treatment at the lowest usual dosage (systemic drugs; cyclosporine and azathioprine cost calculated for a patient weighing 80 kg). WAC = wholesaler acquisition cost or manufacturer's published price to wholesalers; WAC represents a published catalogue or list price and may not represent an actual transactional price. Source: Analy-Source® Monthly. May 5, 2020. Reprinted with permission by First Databank, Inc. All rights reserved. ©2020. www.fdbhealth.com/policies/drug-pricing-policy.
3. If moisturizers are used, they should be applied after the drug. Should not be used with occlusive dressings. Exposure to natural or artificial sunlight should be avoided during treatment. Not recommended for continuous long-term use.

Usual Dosage[1]	Cost[2]
≥2 yrs: apply bid[3]	$500.70 590.10
2-15 yrs: apply 0.03% bid[3] ≥16 yrs: apply 0.03% or 0.1% bid[3]	375.80[4] 562.80[4]
≥3 mos: apply bid	652.20
≥60 kg: 600 mg SC, then 300 mg SC q2 wks 30-59 kg (6-17 yrs): 400 mg SC, then 200 mg SC q2 wks 15-29 kg (6-17 yrs): 600 mg SC, then 300 mg SC q4 wks	10,107.50
2.5-5 mg/kg/day PO in 2 divided doses[6]	672.70 1620.50 1259.30
7.5-25 mg/wk PO in a single dose or in 3 divided doses over 36 hours	50.70
7.5-25 mg SC or IM once/wk 10-25 mg SC once/wk	89.10 2111.90
10-25 mg SC once/wk	1602.30
1-3 mg/kg PO once/day[8]	75.60 1359.80 713.20

4. Both strengths cost the same.
5. Not FDA-approved for treatment of atopic dermatitis.
6. Should not be used continuously for >1 year.
7. Folic acid supplementation is recommended during treatment with methotrexate to reduce the likelihood of hematologic and GI toxicity.
8. Baseline thiopurine methyltransferase (TPMT) testing is recommended before starting therapy; avoid use in patients with very low or absent enzyme activity.

for treatment of patients ≥6 years old with moderate to severe AD that has not responded to topical therapies.[19]

In two randomized, double-blind, 16-week trials in 1379 adults with moderate to severe AD, dupilumab monotherapy significantly improved measures of skin clearing, overall extent and severity of disease, and pruritus compared to placebo. A score of 0 or 1 (clear or almost clear) on the Investigator's Global Assessment (IGA) scale and a ≥2 point reduction from baseline, the primary endpoint, occurred in 38% and 36% of patients treated with dupilumab in the two trials versus 10% and 8% of those who received placebo.[20]

In a randomized, double-blind, 16-week trial in 251 adolescents with moderate to severe AD, a significantly higher percentage of patients achieved an IGA score of 0 or 1 with dupilumab monotherapy than with placebo (24% vs 2%).[21] An unpublished, randomized, double-blind, 16-week trial (summarized in the package insert) compared dupilumab plus topical corticosteroids to topical corticosteroids alone in 367 children 6-11 years old with severe AD; significantly more patients achieved an IGA score of 0 or 1 with addition of dupilumab.

A randomized 52-week trial in adults found that administration of dupilumab in combination with topical corticosteroids significantly improved skin clearing and overall disease severity compared to use of topical corticosteroids alone.[22] Dupilumab plus topical corticosteroids has been shown to be effective in adults with a history of inadequate response to or intolerance of cyclosporine.[23]

Adverse Effects – In AD clinical trials, the incidence of conjunctivitis was higher with dupilumab than with placebo (9-22% vs 2-11%). Ocular surface disorders are common complications of severe atopic dermatitis; the mechanism by which dupilumab might increase the risk is unclear.[24] In a meta-analysis of 8 randomized, controlled trials in adults with moderate to severe AD, dupilumab was associated with a higher risk of injection-site reactions, conjunctivitis, and headache than placebo and a lower risk of skin infection.[25] Development or exacerbation of head and neck dermatitis ("dupilumab facial redness") has been reported in about 10% of AD patients treated with the drug.[26]

Pregnancy and Lactation – Available data from case reports of dupilumab use in pregnant women have not shown a drug-associated risk of major birth defects or adverse maternal or fetal outcomes. No adverse developmental effects were detected in the offspring of monkeys injected with up to 10 times the maximum recommended human dose of another antibody against the IL-4 receptor alpha subunit.

Whether dupilumab is present in human breast milk is unknown, but human IgG is secreted in breast milk. No data are available on the effects of the drug on the breastfed infant or milk production.

CYCLOSPORINE — Oral cyclosporine (*Neoral*, and generics) has been used off-label for treatment of AD that has not responded to topical therapy.[15] In short-term trials, it has decreased AD severity scores by >50% compared to placebo.[17] In a randomized, double-blind trial, significantly more patients with severe AD achieved stable remission with cyclosporine than with prednisolone.[27] A meta-analysis of randomized trials in patients with moderate to severe AD found that cyclosporine and dupilumab were similarly effective for up to 16 weeks of treatment; cyclosporine was superior to methotrexate and azathioprine.[28]

An improvement in disease severity usually occurs within 4 weeks of starting treatment.[17] Cyclosporine should not be used continuously for >1 year.

Adverse Effects – Cyclosporine can cause hypertension, nephrotoxicity, GI disturbances, gingival hyperplasia, hirsutism, headache, paresthesias, hypertriglyceridemia, and musculoskeletal or joint pain. It also increases the risks of infection and cutaneous and lymphoproliferative malignancies, and interacts with many other drugs.

Pregnancy and Lactation – Cyclosporine use during pregnancy has been associated with low birth weight and prematurity. It is present in human breast milk and detectable blood levels have been reported in breastfed infants whose mothers were taking the drug.

METHOTREXATE — Methotrexate taken orally or injected has been used off-label in the treatment of severe refractory AD.[15] No placebo-controlled trials are available, but in a randomized trial in 97 patients with moderate to severe AD, methotrexate 25 mg/week was noninferior to cyclosporine 5 mg/kg/day after 20 weeks of treatment.[29] The time to maximum effect of methotrexate averages 10 weeks.

Adverse Effects – Methotrexate can cause GI adverse effects (particularly with oral administration), fatigue, and aminotransferase elevations. Macrocytic anemia, leukopenia, thrombocytopenia, and hepatic and pulmonary fibrosis can occur. Folic acid supplementation is recommended to reduce the risk of hematologic and GI toxicity.

Pregnancy and Lactation – Methotrexate is contraindicated for use during pregnancy and in women who are breastfeeding.

AZATHIOPRINE — The oral purine analog azathioprine (*Imuran,* and others) has also been used off-label in refractory AD.[15] In a randomized trial in 42 adults with severe AD, methotrexate and azathioprine were equally effective in reducing AD severity scores at 12 weeks.[30] The clinical benefits of azathioprine may not become apparent until ≥12 weeks after starting treatment.

Adverse Effects – GI intolerance, hepatitis, and bone marrow suppression can occur. An increased risk of lymphoma has been reported.

Pregnancy and Lactation – Adverse pregnancy outcomes have been reported in animal studies of azathioprine, but recent data in pregnant women with inflammatory bowel disease suggest that the drug is not associated with adverse birth outcomes.

MYCOPHENOLATE MOFETIL — Mycophenolate mofetil (*Cell-cept,* and others) has been effective in some AD patients with refractory disease, but data are limited. A meta-analysis of studies that included a total of 140 patients with refractory AD treated with mycophenolate mofetil found that 78% reported partial or full remission of AD symptoms. The average time to an initial effect was 7 weeks and the average duration of treatment was 34 weeks.[31] Dosing has ranged from 0.5-3 g/day.

Adverse Effects – Nausea, vomiting, and abdominal cramping are the most common adverse effects of mycophenolate mofetil. Anemia, leukopenia, and thrombocytopenia have been reported rarely.

Pregnancy and Lactation – Use of mycophenolate mofetil during pregnancy has been associated with an increased risk of first-trimester pregnancy loss and congenital malformations. The drug has been detected in the milk of lactating rats. According to limited data from a pregnancy registry, no adverse events were reported in infants who were breastfed for up to 14 months while their mothers were taking mycophenolate mofetil.

ORAL CORTICOSTEROIDS — Oral corticosteroids are FDA-approved for treatment of AD and are frequently prescribed for treatment of moderate to severe disease, but guidelines generally discourage their use, particularly in children. Short courses of an oral corticosteroid can be effective in controlling severe acute exacerbations of AD, but severe rebound of symptoms can occur when the drug is stopped. The dose should be tapered as the drug is discontinued and intensified treatment with topical anti-inflammatory drugs should be started during the taper, but rebound flares may still occur.[32]

ORAL ANTIHISTAMINES — There is no convincing evidence that either first- or second-generation oral antihistamines are effective for treatment of AD.[33] Optimal pruritus control is achieved by regular applications of emollients and topical anti-inflammatory medications.

OTHER DRUGS — The Janus kinase (JAK) signaling pathway is involved in immune-mediated inflammatory skin diseases such as AD, but no JAK inhibitors are currently FDA-approved for treatment of dermatological diseases. The oral JAK inhibitors **tofacitinib** *(Xeljanz, Xeljanz XR)*, **baricitinib** *(Olumiant)*, **upadacitinib** *(Rinvoq)*, and **abrocitinib** (an investigational drug), have been shown to significantly improve AD symptoms compared to placebo.[34-36]

Several biologics are under investigation for use in the treatment of moderate to severe AD. A few case reports suggest that the IL-12 and -23 antagonist **ustekinumab** *(Stelara)* may be effective in some patients with severe AD, but more data are needed.[37] In a randomized, double-blind, 16-week trial in adults with moderate to severe AD, monotherapy with **lebrikizumab**, an investigational IL-13 antagonist, resulted in significant clinical improvement compared to placebo.[38] In a randomized, double-blind, 24-week trial, **nemolizumab**, an investigational antibody against the receptor A of IL-31, which is overexpressed in skin lesions of atopic dermatitis, significantly improved cutaneous signs of inflammation and pruritus compared to placebo in patients with moderate to severe AD.[39]

The oral PDE4 inhibitor **apremilast** *(Otezla)*, which is FDA-approved for treatment of moderate to severe plaque psoriasis and psoriatic arthritis, has markedly improved symptoms in a few patients with severe, refractory AD.[40]

PROBIOTICS — Probiotics have been helpful in some GI disorders[41] and are increasingly being used for treatment of AD. However, a meta-analysis of 39 randomized, controlled trials in 2599 patients (mainly children) with mild to severe AD found that treatment with probiotics (*Lactobacillus* or *Bifidobacteria* species) at varied doses and concentrations for 6 weeks to 3 months did not reduce symptom severity or improve quality of life. Infectious complications, including sepsis, have been reported rarely.[42]

ALLERGEN-SPECIFIC IMMUNOTHERAPY — Subcutaneous and sublingual immunotherapy (SCIT; SLIT) have been shown to be effective for treatment of atopic conditions such as allergic rhinitis and allergic asthma. Small randomized, controlled trials have been conducted in AD patients allergic to environmental allergens; a few showed reductions in disease severity and itching, but others did not. More studies are needed.[43]

1. W Frazier and N Bhardwaj. Atopic dermatitis: diagnosis and treatment. Am Fam Physician 2020; 101:590.
2. R Tanei. Atopic dermatitis in older adults: a review of treatment options. Drugs & Aging 2020; 37:149.
3. EJ van Zuuren et al. Emollients and moisturisers for eczema. Cochrane Database Syst Rev 2017; 2:CD012119.
4. JR Chalmers et al. Daily emollient during infancy for prevention of eczema: the BEEP randomised controlled trial. Lancet 2020; 395:962.
5. L Davallow Gahar et al. Low risk of adrenal insufficiency after use of low- to moderate-potency topical corticosteroids for children with atopic dermatitis. Clin Pediatr (Phila) 2019; 58:406.
6. EC Siegfried et al. Systematic review of published trials: long-term safety of topical corticosteroids and topical calcineurin inhibitors in pediatric patients with atopic dermatitis. BMC Pediatr 2016; 16:75.
7. LF Eichenfield et al. Guidelines of care for the management of atopic dermatitis: section 2. management and treatment of atopic dermatitis with topical therapies. J Am Acad Dermatol 2014; 71:116.
8. JA Broeders et al. Systematic review and meta-analysis of randomized clinical trials (RCTs) comparing topical calcineurin inhibitors with topical corticosteroids for atopic dermatitis: a 15-year experience. J Am Acad Dermatol 2016; 75:410.
9. J Castellsague et al. A cohort study on the risk of lymphoma and skin cancer in users of topical tacrolimus, pimecrolimus, and corticosteroids (Joint European Longitudinal Lymphoma and Skin Cancer Evaluation – JOELLE study). Clin Epidemiol 2018; 10:299.
10. Crisaborole (Eucrisa) for atopic dermatitis. Med Lett Drugs Ther 2017; 59:34.
11. AS Paller et al. Efficacy and safety of crisaborole ointment, a novel, nonsteroidal phosphodiesterase 4 (PDE4) inhibitor for the topical treatment of atopic dermatitis (AD) in children and adults. J Am Acad Dermatol 2016; 75:494.
12. A Ahmed et al. Magnitude of benefit for topical crisaborole in the treatment of atopic dermatitis in children and adults does not look promising: a critical appraisal. Br J Dermatol 2018; 178:659.
13. LF Eichenfield et al. Long-term safety of crisaborole ointment 2% in children and adults with mild to moderate atopic dermatitis. J Am Acad Dermatol 2017; 77:641.
14. J Schlessinger et al. Safety, effectiveness, and pharmacokinetics of crisaborole in infants aged 3 to <24 months with mild-to-moderate atopic dermatitis: a phase IV open-label study (CrisADe CARE 1). Am J Clin Dermatol 2020; 21:275.
15. R Sidbury et al. Guidelines of care for the management of atopic dermatitis: section 3. management and treatment with phototherapy and systemic agents. J Am Acad Dermatol 2014; 71:327.

16. FM Garritsen et al. Photo(chemo)therapy in the management of atopic dermatitis: an updated systematic review with implications for practice and research. Br J Dermatol 2014; 170:501.
17. M Boguniewicz et al. Expert perspectives on management of moderate-to-severe atopic dermatitis: a multidisciplinary consensus addressing current and emerging therapies. J Allergy Clin Immunol Pract 2017; 5:1519.
18. EW Seger et al. Relative efficacy of systemic treatments for atopic dermatitis. J Am Acad Dermatol 2019; 80:411.
19. Dupilumab (Dupixent) for moderate to severe atopic dermatitis. Med Lett Drugs Ther 2017; 59:64.
20. EL Simpson et al. Two phase 3 trials of dupilumab versus placebo in atopic dermatitis. N Engl J Med 2016; 375:2335.
21. EL Simpson et al. Efficacy and safety of dupilumab in adolescents with uncontrolled moderate to severe atopic dermatitis: a phase 3 randomized clinical trial. JAMA Dermatol 2020; 156:44.
22. A Blauvelt et al. Long-term management of moderate-to-severe atopic dermatitis with dupilumab and concomitant topical corticosteroids (LIBERTY AD CHRONOS): a 1-year, randomised, double-blinded, placebo-controlled phase 3 trial. Lancet 2017; 389:2287.
23. M de Bruin-Weller et al. Dupilumab with concomitant topical corticosteroid treatment in adults with atopic dermatitis with an inadequate response or intolerance to ciclosporin A or when this treatment is medically inadvisable: a placebo-controlled, randomized phase III clinical trial (LIBERTY AD CAFÉ). Br J Dermatol 2018; 178:1083.
24. CA Utine et al. Ocular surface disease associated with dupilumab treatment for atopic diseases. Ocul Surf 2020 May 18 (epub).
25. Z Ou et al. Adverse events of dupilumab in adults with moderate-to-severe atopic dermatitis: a meta-analysis. Int Immunopharmacol 2018; 54:303.
26. A Soria et al. Development or exacerbation of head and neck dermatitis in patients treated for atopic dermatitis with dupilumab. JAMA Dermatol 2019; 155:1312.
27. J Schmitt et al. Prednisolone vs. ciclosporin for severe adult eczema. An investigator-initiated double-blind placebo-controlled multicentre trial. Br J Dermatol 2010; 162:661.
28. AM Drucker et al. Systemic immunomodulatory treatments for patients with atopic dermatitis: a systematic review and network meta-analysis. JAMA Dermatol 2020 Apr 22 (epub).
29. C Goujon et al. Methotrexate versus cyclosporine in adults with moderate-to-severe atopic dermatitis: a phase III randomized noninferiority trial. J Allergy Clin Immunol Pract 2018; 6:562.
30. ME Schram et al. A randomized trial of methotrexate versus azathioprine for severe atopic eczema. J Allergy Clin Immunol 2011; 128:353.
31. K Phan and SD Smith. Mycophenolate mofetil and atopic dermatitis: systematic review and meta-analysis. J Dermatolog Treat 2019 Aug 1 (epub).
32. AM Drucker et al. Use of systemic corticosteroids for atopic dermatitis: International Eczema Council consensus statement. Br J Dermatol 2018; 178:768.
33. U Matterne et al. Oral H1 antihistamines as 'add-on' therapy to topical treatment for eczema. Cochrane Database Syst Rev 2019; 1:CD012167.

34. M Napolitano et al. Profile of baricitinib and its potential in the treatment of moderate to severe atopic dermatitis: a short review on the emerging clinical evidence. J Asthma Allergy 2020; 13:89.

35. E Guttman-Yassky et al. Upadacitinib in adults with moderate to severe atopic dermatitis: 16-week results from a randomized, placebo-controlled trial. J Allergy Clin Immunol 2020; 145:877.

36. AM Montilla et al. Scoping review on the use of drugs targeting JAK/STAT pathway in atopic dermatitis, vitiligo, and alopecia areata. Dermatol Ther (Heidelb) 2019; 9:655.

37. D Deleanu and I Nedelea. Biological therapies for atopic dermatitis: an update (review). Exp Ther Med 2019; 17:1061.

38. E Guttman-Yassky et al. Efficacy and safety of lebrikizumab, a high-affinity interleukin 13 inhibitor, in adults with moderate to severe atopic dermatitis: a phase 2b randomized clinical trial. JAMA Dermatol 2020; 156:411.

39. JI Silverberg et al. Phase 2B randomized study of nemolizumab in adults with moderate-to-severe atopic dermatitis and severe pruritus. J Allergy Clin Immunol 2020; 145:173.

40. M Abrouk et al. Apremilast treatment of atopic dermatitis and other chronic eczematous dermatoses. J Am Acad Dermatol 2017; 77:177.

41. Drugs for irritable bowel syndrome. Med Lett Drugs Ther 2020; 62:41.

42. A Makrgeorgou et al. Probiotics for treating eczema. Cochrane Database Syst Rev 2018; 11:CD006135.

43. P Rizk et al. Allergen immunotherapy and atopic dermatitis: the good, the bad, and the unknown. Curr Allergy Asthma Rep 2019; 19:57.

DRUGS FOR
COPD

Original publication date – September 2020

The main goals of treatment for chronic obstructive pulmonary disease (COPD) are to relieve symptoms, reduce the frequency and severity of exacerbations, and prevent disease progression. Several guidelines and review articles on COPD treatment have been published in recent years.[1-5] Treatment of acute exacerbations is not discussed here.

SMOKING CESSATION — Cigarette smoking is the primary cause of COPD in the US. Smoking cessation offers health benefits at all stages of the disease and can slow the decline of lung function. Behavioral modification and pharmacotherapy can help patients stop smoking. Varenicline *(Chantix)* appears to be the most effective drug for treatment of tobacco dependence. Nicotine replacement therapy and bupropion (*Zyban*, and others) are also effective. Combination therapy has been more effective than monotherapy.[6]

VACCINES — Annual vaccination against seasonal influenza can reduce the incidence of acute exacerbations and lower respiratory infections in patients with COPD.[7-9] Pneumococcal vaccines (PCV13 and PPSV23) can reduce the incidence of acute exacerbations and pneumococcal pneumonia. The PPSV23 vaccine is recommended for all patients with COPD. Administration of the PCV13 vaccine is also recommended for those ≥65 years old.[1,10] There should be at least a 1-year interval between the 2 vaccines.

Summary: Drugs for COPD

► Patients with COPD should stop smoking; pharmacotherapy can be helpful.
► Influenza and pneumococcal vaccines decrease the incidence of exacerbations and lower respiratory infections.
► Pulmonary rehabilitation should be considered for all patients.
► All patients should be assessed for proper inhalation technique.
► Patients with occasional dyspnea can use inhaled short-acting bronchodilators as needed for acute symptom relief.
► For patients who have moderate to severe symptoms or a history of exacerbations, regular treatment with an inhaled long-acting bronchodilator (an antimuscarinic or a beta$_2$-agonist) can relieve symptoms, improve lung function, and reduce the frequency of exacerbations.
► Combination therapy with an inhaled long-acting antimuscarinic plus an inhaled long-acting beta$_2$-agonist or an inhaled corticosteroid plus an inhaled long-acting beta$_2$-agonist can be used in patients who are inadequately controlled on monotherapy.
► Triple therapy is recommended for patients with moderate to severe COPD who are not adequately controlled on an inhaled long-acting beta$_2$-agonist plus either an inhaled long-acting antimuscarinic or an inhaled corticosteroid.
► Patients with higher blood eosinophil counts or asthma appear to be the most likely to benefit from addition of an inhaled corticosteroid.
► The oral phosphodiesterase-4 inhibitor roflumilast *(Daliresp)* can be added in patients with chronic bronchitis who continue to have exacerbations on maximal inhaled therapy.
► Addition of the macrolide antibiotic azithromycin (*Zithromax*, and generics) can be considered for patients who are not current smokers who continue to have exacerbations on maximal inhaled therapy.
► Oxygen therapy can improve survival in patients with severe hypoxemia.

PULMONARY REHABILITATION — The benefits of pulmonary rehabilitation programs for patients with COPD are well established. Pulmonary rehabilitation can improve dyspnea, functional capacity, and quality of life, and reduce the number of hospitalizations.[11]

INHALED SHORT-ACTING BRONCHODILATORS — For patients with occasional dyspnea, an inhaled short-acting bronchodilator can provide acute symptom relief. Short-acting drugs, which include inhaled **beta$_2$-agonists** such as albuterol and the **antimuscarinic** ipratropium, can relieve symptoms and improve FEV_1 (forced expiratory volume in one second). Short-acting beta$_2$-agonists have a more rapid onset of action than ipratropium, but ipratropium has a longer duration of action (6-8 hrs vs 3-6 hrs). Combining a short-acting beta$_2$-agonist with ipratropium is more effective than taking either drug alone. The combination of ipratropium and albuterol is available in a single inhaler (see Table 1).

Regular use of an inhaled short-acting bronchodilator is not recommended for treatment of COPD, but patients on maintenance treatment should have a short-acting bronchodilator available for use as needed for acute symptom relief.

INHALED LONG-ACTING BRONCHODILATORS — Regular treatment with an inhaled long-acting bronchodilator (either a beta$_2$-agonist or an antimuscarinic drug) is recommended for patients who have moderate to severe symptoms or a history of exacerbations. As monotherapy, long-acting antimuscarinic agents (LAMAs) have been found to be more effective than long-acting beta$_2$-agonists (LABAs) in preventing exacerbations.[1]

LAMAs — LAMAs have a duration of action of 12-24 hours. They have been shown to improve lung function and reduce exacerbations and hospitalization rates.[12-17] Five inhaled LAMAs are available alone or in fixed-dose combinations with other drugs (see Tables 1 and 3).

Adverse Effects – Inhaled LAMAs have limited systemic absorption. They commonly cause dry mouth. Pharyngeal irritation, urinary retention, and increases in intraocular pressure may occur; antimuscarinic inhalers should be used with caution in patients with narrow-angle glaucoma and in those with symptomatic prostatic hypertrophy or bladder neck obstruction.

Data on the cardiovascular risks of LAMAs in patients with COPD are conflicting; meta-analyses and cohort studies have reported an increased risk of cardiovascular events in patients treated with antimuscarinic agents,[18-21] but results of randomized, controlled trials have not.[22-24]

Table 1. Inhaled Bronchodilators for COPD

Drug	Some Available Formulations
Inhaled Short-Acting Antimuscarinic Agent	
Ipratropium – *Atrovent HFA* (Boehringer Ingelheim)	17 mcg/inh
generic	200 mcg/mL soln
Inhaled Short-Acting Beta$_2$-Agonists[5]	
Albuterol – *ProAir HFA* (Teva)	90 mcg/inh
generic	
Proventil HFA (Merck)	90 mcg/inh
generic	
Ventolin HFA (GSK)	90 mcg/inh
ProAir Respiclick (Teva)	90 mcg/inh
ProAir Digihaler[6] (Teva)	90 mcg/inh
generic	0.63, 1.25, 2.5 mg/3 mL soln
Levalbuterol – *Xopenex HFA* (Sunovion)	45 mcg/inh
Xopenex (Akorn)	0.31, 0.63, 1.25 mg/3 mL soln
generic	
Inhaled Short-Acting Beta$_2$-Agonist/Short-Acting Antimuscarinic Agent Combination	
Albuterol/ipratropium – *Combivent Respimat* (Boehringer Ingelheim)	100 mcg/20 mcg/inh
generic	2.5 mg/0.5 mg/3 mL soln
Inhaled Long-Acting Antimuscarinic Agents (LAMAs)[9]	
Aclidinium – *Tudorza Pressair* (Circassia)	400 mcg/inh
Glycopyrrolate – *Lonhala Magnair* (Sunovion)	25 mcg/mL soln
Revefenacin – *Yupelri* (Mylan)	175 mcg/3 mL

DPI = dry powder inhaler; HFA = hydrofluoroalkane; inh = inhalation; ISI = inhalation spray inhaler; MDI = metered-dose inhaler
1. All patients should be assessed for proper inhalation technique.
2. Approximate WAC for 30 days' treatment at the lowest recommended adult dosage. For short-acting beta$_2$-agonists and *Atrovent HFA*, cost is for 200 inhalations. WAC = wholesaler acquisition cost or manufacturer's published price to wholesalers; WAC represents a published catalogue or list price and may not represent an actual transactional price. Source: AnalySource® Monthly. August 5, 2020. Reprinted with permission by First Databank, Inc. All rights reserved. ©2020. www.fdbhealth.com/policies/drug-pricing-policy.
3. Nebulized solutions may be used for very young, very old, and other patients unable to use handheld inhalers. More time is required to administer the drug and the device may not be portable. Nebulizers and nebulized drugs may be covered as durable medical equipment (DME) under Medicare part B.
4. Cost for 100 doses.

Delivery Device[1]	Usual Adult Dosage	Cost[2]
HFA MDI (200 inh/unit)	2 inh qid PRN	$411.40
Nebulizer[3]	500 mcg qid PRN	17.60[4]
HFA MDI (200 inh/unit)	90-180 mcg q4-6h PRN	66.90
		36.00
HFA MDI (200 inh/unit)	90-180 mcg q4-6h PRN	79.70
		36.00
HFA MDI (60 or 200 inh/unit)	90-180 mcg q4-6h PRN	55.40
DPI (200 inh/unit)	90-180 mcg q4-6h PRN	62.50
DPI (200 inh/unit)	90-180 mcg q4-6h PRN	146.70
Nebulizer[3]	1.25-5 mg q4-8h PRN	17.50[7]
HFA MDI (200 inh/unit)	90 mcg q4-6h PRN	68.20
Nebulizer[3]	0.63-1.25 mg tid PRN	1044.00[4]
		315.50[4]
ISI (120 inh/unit)	1 inh qid PRN	426.50[8]
Nebulizer[3]	2.5 mg/0.5 mg qid PRN	66.90[8]
DPI (30, 60 inh/unit)	1 inh bid	571.50
Nebulizer[3,10]	25 mcg bid	1132.80
Nebulizer[3]	175 mcg once/day[11]	1103.40

5. Not FDA-approved for treatment of COPD.
6. Contains a QR code and a built-in electronic module which automatically detects, records, and stores data on inhaler events such as peak inspiratory flow rate. The device can pair with and transmit data to the mobile app via Bluetooth. The *ProAir Digihaler* contains a lithium-manganese dioxide battery.
7. Cost for 100 2.5-mg doses.
8. Cost for 120 doses.
9. *Seebri Neohaler* (glycopyrrolate), *Utibron Neohaler* (glycopyrrolate/indacaterol), and *Arcapta Neohaler* (indacaterol) are no longer available in the US as of April 1, 2020.
10. Glycopyrrolate inhalation solution should only be used with the *Magnair* handheld nebulizer. Each dose should be administered over a period of 2-3 minutes.
11. Not recommended for use in patients with hepatic impairment. Patients with severe renal impairment (CrCl <30 mL/min) should be monitored for systemic anticholinergic effects.

Continued on next page

Drug	Some Available Formulations
Table 1. Inhaled Bronchodilators for COPD (continued)	
Inhaled Long-Acting Antimuscarinic Agents (LAMAs)[9] (continued)	
Tiotropium –	
Spiriva Handihaler (Boehringer Ingelheim)	18 mcg/cap
Spiriva Respimat	2.5 mcg/inh
Umeclidinium – *Incruse Ellipta* (GSK)	62.5 mcg/inh
Inhaled Long-Acting Beta$_2$-Agonists (LABAs)	
Arformoterol – *Brovana* (Sunovion)	15 mcg/2 mL soln
Formoterol – *Perforomist* (Mylan)	20 mcg/2 mL soln
Olodaterol – *Striverdi Respimat* (Boehringer Ingelheim)	2.5 mcg/inh
Salmeterol – *Serevent Diskus* (GSK)	50 mcg/blister
Inhaled Long-Acting Antimuscarinic Agent/Long-Acting Beta$_2$-Agonist Combinations (LAMA/LA	
Aclidinium/formoterol – *Duaklir Pressair* (Circassia)	400 mcg/12 mcg/inh
Glycopyrrolate/formoterol – *Bevespi Aerosphere* (AstraZeneca)	9 mcg/4.8 mcg/inh
Tiotropium/olodaterol – *Stiolto Respimat* (Boehringer Ingelheim)	2.5 mcg/2.5 mcg/inh
Umeclidinium/vilanterol – *Anoro Ellipta* (GSK)	62.5 mcg/25 mcg/inh

DPI = dry powder inhaler; HFA = hydrofluoroalkane; inh = inhalation; ISI = inhalation spray inhaler; MDI = metered-dose inhaler

LABAs — LABAs can provide sustained bronchodilation for at least 12 hours. They have been shown to reduce the frequency of exacerbations in patients with COPD and improve lung function and quality of life.[25] Several inhaled LABAs are available alone or in fixed-dose combinations with other drugs (see Tables 1 and 3).

Adverse Effects – Inhaled beta$_2$-agonists can cause tachycardia, palpitations, QT interval prolongation, hypokalemia, skeletal muscle tremors and cramping, headache, insomnia, and increases in serum glucose concentrations. Unstable angina and myocardial infarction have been

Delivery Device[1]	Usual Adult Dosage	Cost[2]
DPI (5, 30, 90 inh/unit)	18 mcg[12] once/day	$455.20
ISI (60 inh/unit)	2 inh once/day	455.20
DPI (7, 30 inh/unit)	1 inh once/day	343.80
Nebulizer[3]	15 mcg bid	1072.80
Nebulizer[3]	20 mcg bid	1041.00
ISI (60 inh/unit)	2 inh once/day	224.50
DPI (28, 60 inh/unit)	1 inh bid	399.20
Combinations)[9]		
DPI (30, 60 inh/unit)	1 inh bid	995.00
HFA MDI (120 inh/unit)	2 inh bid	383.60
ISI (60 inh/unit)	2 inh once/day	421.50
DPI (7, 30 inh/unit)	1 inh once/day	421.90

12. Contents of one capsule; two inhalations of the powder are required to deliver the full dose.

reported. Tolerance can develop with continued use. LABA monotherapy has been associated with an increased risk of asthma-related death; there is no evidence to date that patients with COPD have a similar risk.

Long-Acting Bronchodilator Combinations – Dual bronchodilator therapy is more effective than monotherapy; it is recommended for patients who are inadequately controlled on a single drug.[26] Combining a LAMA with a LABA can improve lung function and reduce symptoms, and may decrease exacerbation rates in patients with COPD.[27,28] Four fixed-dose LAMA/LABA combinations are available (see Table 1).

Table 2. Long-Acting Bronchodilator Inhalers: Ease of Use*

Aerosphere Inhalers

Bevespi Aerosphere (glycopyrrolate/formoterol), Breztri Aerosphere (budesonide/glycopyrrolate/formoterol fumarate)
- ► Metered-dose inhaler; requires coordination of inhalation with hand-actuation; drug delivery is dependent on ability to perform a slow, deep inhalation
- ► Easy to assemble; requires priming
- ► Indicator shows approximately how many doses are left
- ► Twice-daily dosing

Diskus Inhalers

Advair Diskus (fluticasone propionate/salmeterol), Serevent Diskus (salmeterol)
- ► Dry powder inhaler; drug delivery to lungs is dependent upon ability to perform a rapid, deep inhalation
- ► Indicator shows how many doses are left
- ► Twice-daily dosing

Ellipta Inhalers

Anoro Ellipta (umeclidinium/vilanterol), Breo Ellipta (fluticasone furoate/vilanterol), Incruse Ellipta (umeclidinium), Trelegy Ellipta (fluticasone furoate/umeclidinium/vilanterol)
- ► Dry powder inhaler; drug delivery to lungs is dependent upon ability to perform a long, steady, and deep inhalation
- ► No assembly or priming required
- ► Indicator shows how many doses are left
- ► Doses may be wasted if inhaler is opened/closed accidentally
- ► Once-daily dosing

Handihaler Inhaler

Spiriva Handihaler (tiotropium)
- ► Dry powder inhaler; drug delivery to lungs is dependent upon ability to perform a rapid, deep inhalation
- ► Inserting capsules into the device may be difficult for some patients
- ► Once-daily dosing

*Additional instructions for inhaler use can be found in the online table Correct Use of Inhalers for COPD. Available at: http://secure.medicalletter.org/TML-article-1606e. Accessed August 27, 2020.

Continued on next page

Table 2. Long-Acting Bronchodilator Inhalers: Ease of Use*
(continued)

Pressair **Inhalers**

Duaklir Pressair **(aclidinium/formoterol),** *Tudorza Pressair* **(aclidinium)**
- ▸ Dry powder inhaler; drug delivery to lungs is dependent upon ability to perform a strong, deep inhalation
- ▸ No assembly required
- ▸ Twice-daily dosing

Respiclick **Inhaler**

AirDuo Respiclick **(fluticasone propionate/salmeterol)**
- ▸ Dry powder inhaler; drug delivery to lungs is dependent upon ability to perform a rapid, deep inhalation
- ▸ Indicator shows how many doses are left
- ▸ Doses may be wasted if inhaler is opened/closed accidentally
- ▸ Twice-daily dosing

Respimat **Inhalers**

Spiriva Respimat **(tiotropium),** *Stiolto Respimat* **(tiotropium/olodaterol),**
Striverdi Respimat **(olodaterol)**
- ▸ Inhalation spray inhaler; drug delivery to lungs is not dependent on strength of breath intake
- ▸ Assembly may be difficult for some patients
- ▸ Indicator shows approximately how many doses are left
- ▸ Once-daily dosing

*Additional instructions for inhaler use can be found in the online table Correct Use of Inhalers for COPD. Available at: http://secure.medicalletter.org/TML-article-1606e. Accessed August 27, 2020.

INHALED CORTICOSTEROIDS (ICSs) — ICSs should not be used as monotherapy for treatment of COPD. Use of an ICS in addition to a LABA can modestly improve lung function and reduce exacerbations.[29] Addition of an ICS is recommended for patients with moderate to very severe COPD who continue to have exacerbations while receiving long-acting bronchodilators, especially those with blood eosinophil counts ≥300 cells/mcL (patients with levels <100 cells/mcL are less likely to respond) or asthma. Various fixed-dose combinations of ICSs and LABAs are available (see Table 3).

Drugs for COPD

Table 3. Inhaled Corticosteroids and Corticosteroid/Bronchodilator Combinations for COPD

Drug	Some Available Formulations
Inhaled Corticosteroids (ICSs)[3,4]	
Beclomethasone dipropionate – QVAR Redihaler (Teva)	40, 80 mcg/inh
Budesonide[6] – Pulmicort Flexhaler (AstraZeneca)	90, 180 mcg/inh
Ciclesonide – Alvesco (Covis)	80, 160 mcg/inh
Fluticasone furoate – Arnuity Ellipta (GSK)	100, 200 mcg/inh
Fluticasone propionate – Flovent Diskus (GSK)	50, 100, 250 mcg/blister
Flovent HFA (GSK)	44, 110, 220 mcg/inh
ArmonAir Respiclick (Teva)	55, 113, 232 mcg/inh
ArmonAir Digihaler[7] (Teva)	55, 113, 232 mcg/inh
Mometasone furoate –	
Asmanex HFA (Merck)	50, 100, 200 mcg/inh
Asmanex Twisthaler (Merck)	110, 220 mcg/inh
Inhaled Corticosteroid/Long-Acting Beta₂-Agonist Combinations (ICS/LABA Combinations)	
Fluticasone propionate/salmeterol –	
Advair Diskus[8] (GSK) Wixela Inhub[8,10] (Mylan)	100, 250, 500 mcg/50 mcg/ blister
Advair HFA[3] (GSK)	45, 115, 230 mcg/21 mcg/inh
AirDuo Respiclick[3] (Teva) generic[3,11]	55, 113, 232 mcg/14 mcg/inh
AirDuo Digihaler[3,7] (Teva)	55, 113, 232 mcg/14 mcg/inh

DPI = dry powder inhaler; HFA = hydrofluoroalkane; inh = inhalation; ISI = inhalation spray inhaler; MDI = metered-dose inhaler
1. All patients should be assessed for proper inhalation technique.
2. Approximate WAC for 30 days' treatment at the lowest usual adult dosage. WAC = wholesaler acquisition cost or manufacturer's published price to wholesalers; WAC represents a published catalogue or list price and may not represent an actual transactional price. Source: AnalySource® Monthly. August 5, 2020. Reprinted with permission by First Databank, Inc. All rights reserved. ©2020. www.fdbhealth.com/policies/drug-pricing-policy.
3. Not FDA-approved for treatment of COPD.
4. Inhaled corticosteroid monotherapy is not recommended for treatment of COPD.
5. The Redihaler is a breath-actuated MDI that does not require coordination of inhalation with hand-actuation.

Delivery Device[1]	Usual Adult Dosage	Cost[2]
HFA MDI[5] (120 inh/unit)	40-320 mcg bid	$190.20
DPI (60, 120 inh/unit)	180-720 mcg bid	248.20
HFA MDI (60 inh/unit)	80-320 mcg bid	274.20
DPI (14, 30 inh/unit)	100-200 mcg once/day	178.80
DPI (28, 60 inh/unit)	100-1000 mcg bid	192.80
HFA MDI (120 inh/unit)	88-880 mcg bid	192.80
DPI (60 inh/unit)	55-232 mcg bid	169.30
DPI (60 inh/unit)	55-232 mcg bid	299.00[13]
HFA MDI (120 inh/unit)	200-400 mcg bid	224.90
DPI (30, 60, 120 inh/unit)	220-880 mcg once/day in evening or 220 mcg bid	191.60
DPI (28, 60 inh/unit)[9]	250/50 mcg bid	393.90
		116.40
HFA MDI (60, 120 inh/unit)	2 inh bid	317.10
DPI (60 inh/unit)	1 inh bid	320.20
		95.40
DPI (60 inh/unit)	1 inh bid	399.00[12,15]

6. Budesonide is also available as a suspension for nebulization (*Pulmicort Respules*, and generics) that is FDA-approved only for treatment of asthma in children 1-8 years old.
7. Contains a QR code and a built-in electronic module which automatically detects, records, and stores data on inhaler events such as peak inspiratory flow rate. The device can pair with and transmit data to the mobile app via Bluetooth. The *ArmonAir Digihaler* and *AirDuo Digihaler* contain a lithium-manganese dioxide battery.
8. Only the 250/50 mcg dose is FDA-approved for use in COPD.
9. *Wixela Inhub* is only available in 60 inh/unit.
10. Generic equivalent for *Advair Diskus*.
11. Authorized generic.
12. Expected to be available in 2020 in select healthcare systems.

Continued on next page

Table 3. Inhaled Corticosteroids and Corticosteroid/Bronchodilator Combinations for COPD (continued)	
Drug	**Some Available Formulations**
Inhaled Corticosteroid/Long-Acting Beta$_2$-Agonist Combinations (ICS/LABA Combinations) (continued)	
Fluticasone furoate/vilanterol – Breo Ellipta[13] (GSK)	100, 200 mcg/25 mcg/inh
Budesonide/formoterol – generic[11] Symbicort[14] (AstraZeneca)	80, 160 mcg/4.5 mcg/inh
Inhaled Corticosteroid/Long-Acting Antimuscarinic Agent/Long-Acting Beta$_2$-Agonist Combinations (ICS/LAMA/LABA Combinations)	
Budesonide/glycopyrrolate/formoterol fumarate – Breztri Aerosphere (AstraZeneca)	160 mcg/9 mcg/4.8 mcg/inh
Fluticasone furoate/umeclidinium/ vilanterol – Trelegy Ellipta (GSK)	100 mcg/62.5 mcg/25 mcg/inh

DPI = dry powder inhaler; HFA = hydrofluoroalkane; inh = inhalation; ISI = inhalation spray inhaler; MDI = metered-dose inhaler
13. Only the 100/25 mcg dose is FDA-approved for use in COPD.

Adverse Effects – Local adverse effects of ICSs include candidiasis and dysphonia. Systemic absorption of ICSs can cause skin bruising, cataracts, reduced bone mineral density, and an increased risk of fractures. Use of ICSs in patients with COPD has been associated with an increased risk of pneumonia.[30]

LAMA/LABA vs ICS/LABA — In a 52-week, randomized, controlled trial (FLAME) in 1680 patients with COPD, those who received a LAMA/LABA combination had 11% fewer exacerbations, a longer time to the first exacerbation, and a lower incidence of pneumonia than those who received an ICS/LABA combination. The rates of mortality and other adverse effects were similar in the two groups.[31] In a cohort study including 3954 patients, the incidence of exacerbations was similar with a LAMA/LABA and an ICS/LABA combination, but the incidence of pneumonia was lower with the LAMA/LABA combination.[32] In the

Delivery Device[1]	Usual Adult Dosage	Cost[2]
DPI (14, 30 inh/unit)	1 inh once/day	$361.80
HFA MDI (60, 120 inh/unit)	2 inh bid	250.10
		364.40
HFA MDI (28, 120 inh/unit)	2 inh bid	590.40
DPI (14, 30 inh/unit)	1 inh once/day	573.20

14. Only the 160/4.5 mcg dose is FDA-approved for use in COPD.
15. Price accessed October 5, 2020.

randomized, controlled IMPACT trial comparing LAMA/LABA, ICS/LABA, and triple therapy, the annual rate of moderate or severe exacerbations was lower with ICS/LABA therapy than with a LAMA/LABA combination.[33] In all 3 studies, patients with higher blood eosinophil counts were the most likely to benefit from an ICS/LABA combination.

TRIPLE-THERAPY REGIMENS — Adding a third drug can reduce exacerbations and improve lung function, symptoms, and quality of life.

In two randomized controlled trials (IMPACT, TRIBUTE), treatment with two different single-inhaler triple combinations (ICS/LAMA/LABA) modestly decreased the number of COPD exacerbations compared to LAMA/LABA therapy.[33,34] In a post-hoc analysis of results from the IMPACT trial, all-cause mortality was significantly lower with triple therapy (2.36%) than with a LAMA/LABA combination (3.19%).[35]

Table 4. Other Drugs for COPD	
Drug	**Some Available Formulations**
Phosphodiesterase-4 (PDE4) Inhibitor	
Roflumilast − *Daliresp* (AstraZeneca)	250, 500 mcg tabs
Macrolide Antibiotic	

Azithromycin[3] − generic
  Zithromax (Pfizer)
	250, 500, 600 mg tabs; 100 mg/5 mL,
	  200 mg/5 mL susp

Methylxanthine	
Theophylline[4,5] − generic	100, 200, 300, 400, 450, 600 mg ER tabs; 80 mg/15 mL soln
Elixophyllin (Nostrum Labs)	80 mg/15 mL soln
Theo-24 (Auxilium)	100, 200, 300, 400 mg ER caps

ER = extended release; soln = solution; susp = suspension
1 Approximate WAC for 30 days' treatment at the lowest usual adult dosage. WAC = wholesaler acquisition cost or manufacturer's published price to wholesalers; WAC represents a published catalogue or list price and may not represent an actual transactional price. Source: AnalySource® Monthly. August 5, 2020. Reprinted with permission by First Databank, Inc. All rights reserved. ©2020. www.fdbhealth.com/policies/drug-pricing-policy.

A randomized controlled trial (ETHOS) compared triple therapy with low-dose ICS (budesonide 160 mcg), triple therapy with high-dose ICS (budesonide 320 mcg), dual therapy with a LAMA/LABA combination, and dual therapy with a LABA/high-dose ICS combination in 8509 patients with moderate to very severe COPD. Both ICS triple therapy regimens reduced the annual rate of moderate to severe exacerbations compared to dual therapy. High-dose ICS triple therapy significantly reduced overall mortality compared to LAMA/LABA dual therapy, but low-dose ICS triple therapy did not. The incidence of pneumonia was higher with ICS-containing regimens than with the LAMA/LABA regimen.[36]

Two fixed-dose inhalers containing an ICS, LAMA, and LABA are available (see Table 3).

ICS DISCONTINUATION — In one study, 2485 patients with COPD on triple therapy were randomized to either continue triple therapy or

Usual Adult Dosage	Cost[1]
500 mcg PO once/day[2]	$382.90
250 mg PO once/day or 500 mg three times/week	56.80
	63.80
300-600 mg PO once/day or divided bid	15.80
300-600 mg/day PO divided tid-qid	1261.30
300-600 mg PO once/day[6]	82.20

2. Usual maintenance dosage. Recommended starting dosage is 250 mcg once/day for 4 weeks.
3. Not FDA-approved for treatment of COPD.
4. Extended-release formulations may not be interchangeable.
5. Periodic monitoring is recommended to maintain peak serum concentrations between 6 and 12 mcg/mL.
6. *Theo-24* should not be taken <1 hr before a high-fat content meal; the entire 24-hour dose can be released in a 4-hour period, resulting in toxicity.

taper the ICS over 12 weeks. The time to the first moderate or severe exacerbation within 12 months was similar in both groups, but a statistically significant decrease in trough FEV_1 occurred in the ICS taper group; the clinical significance is unclear.[37] A post-hoc analysis found that the risk of exacerbation was significantly higher in the ICS taper group compared to the continuation group in patients who had blood eosinophil levels ≥300 cells/mcL at baseline.[38] In another study, 527 patients with moderate to severe COPD who were on long-term triple therapy without frequent exacerbations were randomized to continue triple therapy or switch to LAMA/LABA dual therapy. A significant reduction in trough FEV_1 occurred in the ICS withdrawal group, and patients with blood eosinophil levels >300 cells/mcL had a higher risk of exacerbations.[39]

ROFLUMILAST—Roflumilast *(Daliresp)* is an oral phosphodiesterase-4 (PDE4) inhibitor FDA-approved for use in patients with severe COPD associated with chronic bronchitis and a history of exacerbations. It reduces inflammation by increasing intracellular levels of cAMP; it does

Table 5. Treatment of COPD[1,2]

Occasional Dyspnea or Other Symptoms; ≤1 exacerbation[3]

	Inhaled ipratropium as needed
or	Inhaled short-acting beta₂-agonist as needed
or	LAMA
or	LABA

Moderate-Severe Dyspnea or Other Symptoms; ≤1 exacerbation[3]

Initial	LAMA
or	LABA
Persistent or Severe Symptoms	LAMA + LABA

Occasional Dyspnea or Other Symptoms; ≥1 exacerbations[4]

Initial	LAMA
Further Exacerbations	LAMA + LABA
or	ICS + LABA[5]

Moderate-Severe Dyspnea or Other Symptoms; ≥1 exacerbations[4]

Initial	LAMA
or	LAMA + LABA
or	ICS + LABA[5]
Further Exacerbations	ICS + LABA + LAMA
or	ICS + LABA + LAMA + roflumilast[6]
or	ICS + LABA + LAMA + azithromycin[7]

ICS = inhaled corticosteroid; LABA = inhaled long-acting beta₂-agonist; LAMA = inhaled long-acting antimuscarinic agent
1. Adapted from the Global Strategy for the Diagnosis, Management, and Prevention of COPD, Global Initiative for Chronic Obstructive Pulmonary Disease (GOLD) 2020. Available at: http://goldcopd.org. Accessed August 27, 2020. Dyspnea and symptoms should be assessed using mMRC (Modified British Medical Research Council) and CAT (COPD Assessment Test), respectively.
2. Short-acting anticholinergics and beta₂-agonists can be added to any regimen for acute relief.
3. Exacerbation that did not lead to hospital admission.
4. ≥1 exacerbation leading to hospital admission or ≥2 exacerbations.
5. An ICS/LABA combination may be considered a first choice for patients with asthma/COPD overlap, blood eosinophil levels ≥300 cells/mcL, or blood eosinophil levels ≥100 cells/mcL and either ≥2 moderate exacerbations or ≥1 hospitalization for exacerbation.
6. In patients with FEV₁ <50% predicted and chronic bronchitis.
7. Or another macrolide. Consider use in patients who are not current smokers.

not cause bronchodilation.[40] Once-daily treatment with roflumilast can modestly improve lung function and reduce the frequency of exacerbations, but it does not appear to improve symptoms or quality of life.[41,42]

Adverse Effects – Common adverse effects include nausea and diarrhea. Significant weight loss and changes in mood and behavior have been reported.

Drug Interactions – Roflumilast is metabolized by CYP3A4 and 1A2; drugs that are inhibitors of CYP3A4 or inhibit both CYP3A4 and 1A2, such as cimetidine, erythromycin, ketoconazole and fluvoxamine, can increase concentrations of roflumilast.[43] Strong inducers of cytochrome P450 enzymes, such as rifampin and carbamazepine, can reduce the efficacy of roflumilast and should be avoided.

AZITHROMYCIN — Macrolide antibiotics have anti-inflammatory effects. Once-daily or three-times-weekly off-label use of azithromycin (*Zithromax*, and generics) has been shown to reduce the risk of exacerbations over one year and improve quality of life in patients with COPD who continue to have exacerbations, especially those who are not current smokers.[44,45]

Adverse Effects – Azithromycin use has been associated with hearing loss, QT interval prolongation, and development of antimicrobial resistance.

Drug Interactions – Use with other drugs that prolong the QT interval can result in additive effects.[46] Azithromycin may increase the risk of toxicity with digoxin, cyclosporine, and tacrolimus.

THEOPHYLLINE — The primary mechanism of action of theophylline is bronchodilation; at low concentrations, it may have anti-inflammatory effects.[47] It does not appear to reduce the risk of exacerbations and is generally not recommended for treatment of COPD.[48] Theophylline has a narrow therapeutic index; periodic monitoring is warranted to maintain peak serum concentrations between 6 and 12 mcg/mL.

Adverse Effects – Dose-related adverse effects of theophylline include nausea, nervousness, headache, and insomnia. Vomiting, hypokalemia, hyperglycemia, tachycardia, cardiac arrhythmias, tremors, neuromuscular irritability, and seizures can occur at supratherapeutic serum concentrations.

Drug Interactions – Theophylline is metabolized hepatically, primarily by CYP1A2 and 3A4; any drug that inhibits or induces these enzymes can affect theophylline serum concentrations.[43]

OXYGEN THERAPY — In patients with severe hypoxemia, use of long-term supplemental oxygen therapy can increase survival and may improve quality of life.[49] In one study, long-term oxygen therapy did not reduce mortality or prolong time to first hospitalization in patients with mild to moderate hypoxemia.[50]

LOW-DOSE MORPHINE — In a randomized, double-blind trial in 124 COPD patients with moderate to very severe breathlessness despite pharmacologic therapy and pulmonary rehabilitation, 4 weeks of treatment with 10 mg of sustained-release morphine twice daily improved breathlessness compared to placebo only in those with severe dyspnea; there was no significant difference between the groups in arterial $PaCO_2$.[51,52]

1. GOLD. Global strategy for the diagnosis, management and prevention of COPD 2020 report. Available at www.goldcopd.org. Accessed August 27, 2020.
2. L Nici et al. Pharmacologic management of chronic obstructive pulmonary disease. An official American Thoracic Society clinical practice guideline. Am J Respir Crit Care Med 2020; 201:e56.
3. BR Celli and JA Wedzicha. Update on clinical aspects of chronic obstructive pulmonary disease. N Engl J Med 2019; 381:1257.
4. CM Riley and FC Sciurba. Diagnosis and outpatient management of chronic obstructive pulmonary disease: a review. JAMA 2019; 321:786.
5. WW Labaki and SR Rosenberg. Chronic obstructive pulmonary disease. Ann Intern Med 2020;173:ITC17.
6. Drugs for smoking cessation. Med Lett Drugs Ther 2019; 61:105.
7. Influenza vaccine for 2019-2020. Med Lett Drugs Ther 2019; 61:161.
8. S Mulpuru et al. Effectiveness of influenza vaccination on hospitalizations and risk factors for severe outcomes in hospitalized patients with COPD. Chest 2019; 155:69.
9. F Froes et al. Pneumococcal vaccination and chronic respiratory diseases. Int J Chron Obstruct Pulmon Dis 2017; 12:3457.
10. CDC. Pneumococcal vaccine timing for adults. June 25, 2020. Available at: www.cdc. gov/pneumococcal/vaccination.html. Accessed August 27, 2020.
11. B McCarthy et al. Pulmonary rehabilitation for chronic obstructive pulmonary disease. Cochrane Database Syst Rev 2015; 2:CD003793.

12. DP Tashkin et al. A 4-year trial of tiotropium in chronic obstructive pulmonary disease. N Engl J Med 2008; 359:1543.
13. M Decramer et al. Effect of tiotropium on outcomes in patients with moderate chronic obstructive pulmonary disease (UPLIFT): a prespecified subgroup analysis of a randomised controlled trial. Lancet 2009; 374:1171.
14. Aclidinium bromide (Tudorza Pressair) for COPD. Med Lett Drugs Ther 2012; 54:99.
15. Seebri Neohaler and Utibron Neohaler for COPD. Med Lett Drugs Ther 2016; 58:39.
16. Umeclidinium (Incruse Ellipta) for COPD. Med Lett Drugs Ther 2015; 57:63.
17. Revefenacin (Yupelri) for COPD. Med Lett Drugs Ther 2019; 61:14.
18. S Singh et al. Inhaled anticholinergics and risk of major adverse cardiovascular events in patients with chronic obstructive pulmonary disease: a systematic review and meta-analysis. JAMA 2008; 300:1439.
19. K MC Verhamme et al. Use of tiotropium Respimat soft mist inhaler versus Handihaler and mortality in patients with COPD. Eur Respir J 2013; 42:606.
20. S Singh et al. Mortality associated with tiotropium mist inhaler in patients with chronic obstructive pulmonary disease: systematic review and meta-analysis of randomised controlled trials. BMJ 2011; 342:d3215.
21. MT Wang et al. Association of cardiovascular risk with inhaled long-acting bronchodilators in patients with chronic obstructive pulmonary disease: a nested case-control study. JAMA Intern Med 2018; 178:229.
22. B Celli et al. Cardiovascular safety of tiotropium in patients with COPD. Chest 2010; 137:20.
23. RA Wise et al. Tiotropium Respimat inhaler and the risk of death in COPD. N Engl J Med 2013; 369:1491.
24. RA Wise et al. Effect of aclidinium bromide on major cardiovascular events and exacerbations in high-risk patients with chronic obstructive pulmonary disease: the ASCENT-COPD randomized clinical trial. JAMA 2019; 321:1693.
25. KM Kew et al. Long-acting beta2-agonists for chronic obstructive pulmonary disease. Cochrane Database Syst Rev 2013; 10:CD010177.
26. M Lipari et al. Dual- versus mono-bronchodilator therapy in moderate to severe COPD: a meta-analysis. Annals Pharmacother 2020; 54:1232.
27. HA Farne and CJ Cates. Long-acting beta2-agonist in addition to tiotropium versus either tiotropium or long-acting beta2-agonist alone for chronic obstructive pulmonary disease. Cochrane Database Syst Rev 2015; 10:CD008989.
28. H Ni et al. Combined aclidinium bromide and long-acting beta2-agonist for chronic obstructive pulmonary disease (COPD). Cochrane Database Syst Rev 2018; 12:CD011594.
29. LJ Nannini et al. Combined corticosteroid and long-acting beta(2)-agonist in one inhaler versus long-acting beta(2)-agonists for chronic obstructive pulmonary disease. Cochrane Database Syst Rev 2012; 9:CD006829.
30. KM Kew and A Seniukovich. Inhaled steroids and risk of pneumonia for chronic obstructive pulmonary disease. Cochrane Database Syst Rev 2014; 3:CD010115.
31. JA Wedzicha et al. Indacaterol-glycopyrronium versus salmeterol-fluticasone for COPD. N Engl J Med 2016; 374:2222.
32. S Suissa et al. Comparative effectiveness and safety of LABA-LAMA vs LABA-ICS treatment of COPD in real-world clinical practice. Chest 2019; 155:1158.

33. DA Lipson et al. Once-daily single-inhaler triple versus dual therapy in patients with COPD. N Engl J Med 2018; 378:1671.
34. A Papi et al. Extrafine inhaled triple therapy versus dual bronchodilatortherapy in chronic obstructive pulmonary disease (TRIBUTE): a double-blind, parallel group, randomized controlled trial. Lancet 2018; 391:1076.
35. DA Lipson et al. Reduction in all-cause mortality with fluticasone furoate/umeclidinium/ vilanterol in patients with chronic obstructive pulmonary disease. Am J Respir Crit Care Med 2020; 201:1508.
36. KF Rabe et al. Triple inhaled therapy at two glucocorticoid doses in moderate-to-very-severe COPD. N Engl J Med 2020; 383:35.
37. H Magnussen et al. Withdrawal of inhaled glucocorticoids and exacerbations of COPD. N Engl J Med 2014; 371:1285.
38. H Watz et al. Blood eosinophil count and exacerbations in severe chronic obstructive pulmonary disease after withdrawal of inhaled corticosteroids: a post-hoc analysis of the WISDOM trial. Lancet Respir Med 2016; 4:390.
39. KR Chapman et al. Long-term triple therapy de-escalation to indacaterol/glycopyrronium in patients with chronic obstructive pulmonary disease (SUNSET): a randomized, double-blind, triple-dummy clinical trial. Am J Respir Crit Care Med 2018; 198:329.
40. Roflumilast (Daliresp) for COPD. Med Lett Drugs Ther 2011; 53:59.
41. PMA Calverley et al. Roflumilast in symptomatic chronic obstructive pulmonary disease: two randomised clinical trials. Lancet 2009; 374:685.
42. J Chong et al. Phosphodiesterase 4 inhibitors for chronic obstructive pulmonary disease. Cochrane Database Syst Rev 2013; 11:CD002309.
43. Inhibitors and inducers of CYP enzymes and P-glycoprotein. Med Lett Drugs Ther 2019 November 6 (epub). Available at: medicalletter.org/downloads/CYP_PGP_Tables.pdf.
44. RK Albert et al. Azithromycin for prevention of exacerbations of COPD. N Engl J Med 2011; 365:689.
45. S Uzun et al. Azithromycin maintenance treatment in patients with frequent exacerbations of chronic obstructive pulmonary disease (COLUMBUS): a randomised, double-blind, placebo-controlled trial. Lancet Respir Med 2014; 2:361.
46. RL Woosley et al. QT drugs list. Available at: www.crediblemeds.org. Accessed August 27, 2020.
47. PJ Barnes. Theophylline. Am J Respir Crit Care Med 2013; 188:901.
48. G Devereux et al. Effect of theophylline as adjunct to inhaled corticosteroids on exacerbations in patients with COPD: a randomized clinical trial. JAMA 2018; 320:1548.
49. JK Stoller et al. Oxygen therapy for patients with COPD: current evidence and the long-term oxygen treatment trial. CHEST 2010; 138:179.
50. Long-Term Oxygen Treatment Trial Research Group et al. A randomized trial of long-term oxygen for COPD with moderate desaturation. N Engl J Med 2016; 375:1617.
51. CA Verberkt et al. Effect of sustained-release morphine for refractory breathlessness in chronic obstructive pulmonary disease on health status: a randomized clinical trial. JAMA Intern Med 2020 August 17 (epub).
52. EW Widera. The role of opioids in patients with chronic obstructive pulmonary disease and chronic breathlessness. JAMA Intern Med 2020 August 17 (epub).

Corticosteroids in Community-Acquired Pneumonia

Original publication date – January 2020

Recently updated guidelines from the American Thoracic Society (ATS) and the Infectious Diseases Society of America (IDSA) address the use of corticosteroids as an adjunct to antimicrobials for treatment of community-acquired pneumonia (CAP).[1]

CLINICAL STUDIES — Severe CAP – Data showing a clinically significant mortality benefit of corticosteroids in the treatment of patients with severe CAP are limited. Some meta-analyses have found a reduced risk of death with corticosteroid use in such patients,[2-4] but others have not,[5,6] and the studies included in the meta-analyses varied in their quality and their definitions of severe CAP.

In one double-blind trial, 46 patients with severe CAP were randomized to receive IV hydrocortisone (200-mg bolus, then 10 mg/hr) or placebo for 7 days in addition to standard treatment. Treatment with hydrocortisone compared to placebo resulted in significantly shorter median durations of mechanical ventilation (4 vs 10 days) and hospital stay (13 vs 21 days). Seven patients in the placebo group died versus none in the hydrocortisone group.[7]

Reductions in the durations of mechanical ventilation and hospital stay also occurred with use of IV hydrocortisone compared to placebo in a single-blind trial in 80 ICU patients with CAP, but baseline serum

Summary: Corticosteroids in CAP

▶ Clinical trials evaluating whether adjunctive use of corticosteroids improves rates of morbidity and mortality in severe CAP have produced mixed results.
▶ There is no evidence that adjunctive use of corticosteroids improves outcomes in mild to moderate CAP.
▶ Corticosteroids increase the risk of hyperglycemia, and their use has been associated with increased rates of bleeding, secondary infection, and rehospitalization.
▶ Guidelines advise against adjunctive treatment of CAP or influenza pneumonia with corticosteroids except in patients with other indications for their use.

creatinine and blood urea nitrogen levels were higher in the placebo group.[8] Chronic kidney disease is associated with an increased risk of pneumonia-related morbidity and mortality.[9]

In another double-blind trial, 785 patients hospitalized with CAP were randomized to receive oral prednisone 50 mg or placebo once daily for 7 days. Time to clinical stability, the primary endpoint, was significantly shorter with prednisone than with placebo (3.0 vs 4.4 days), but prednisone did not significantly improve other clinical outcomes such as mortality rates and pneumonia recurrence, and it significantly increased the risk of hyperglycemia (19% vs 11%). Whether the difference in the primary endpoint shows a real beneficial effect of prednisone or is an artifact of its effects on certain markers of clinical stability (e.g., temperature, blood pressure) is unclear.[10]

In another double-blind trial, 120 patients with severe CAP and a high inflammatory response (C-reactive protein >150 mg/L) were randomized to receive IV methylprednisolone 0.5 mg/kg or placebo every 12 hours for 5 days. Treatment failure, the primary endpoint, occurred significantly less often with methylprednisolone than with placebo (13% vs 31%). This difference was primarily due to a lower rate of late radiographic progression with methylprednisolone (2% vs 15%); the drug did not significantly reduce in-hospital mortality, time to clinical stability, or length of stay.[11]

Mild to Moderate CAP – There is no evidence that corticosteroids reduce mortality rates or other adverse clinical outcomes in patients with mild to moderate CAP. In a randomized, double-blind trial in 816 hospitalized patients with CAP of varying severity, a bundled intervention including use of prednisolone acetate 50 mg/day for 7 days did not improve length of stay, mortality rates, or readmission rates compared to standard treatment and was associated with an increased risk of GI bleeding (2.2% vs 0.7%).[12]

ADVERSE EFFECTS — Hyperglycemia occurs commonly with use of corticosteroids and can be clinically significant.[3,5] Corticosteroids also have been associated with increased rates of bleeding, secondary infection, and rehospitalization.[5,12,13] One meta-analysis found an increased risk of death with use of corticosteroids in small retrospective studies of patients with influenza pneumonia.[14]

GUIDELINES — The new ATS/IDSA guidelines advise against adjunctive corticosteroid treatment of CAP or influenza pneumonia except in patients who have other indications for their use, such as asthma, COPD, or an autoimmune disease. They do endorse the recommendation in current sepsis guidelines that IV hydrocortisone 200 mg/day be used in patients who have CAP with septic shock that is refractory to fluid resuscitation and vasopressor support, even though the sepsis guidelines classify this recommendation as weak and the quality of evidence supporting it as low.[15]

CONCLUSION — Data on whether adjunctive corticosteroids improve clinical outcomes in patients with severe community-acquired pneumonia (CAP) are mixed; until more evidence becomes available, they probably should not be used routinely, but they should be used in patients with refractory septic shock. Corticosteroids can cause clinically significant hyperglycemia. There are no data to support their use in the treatment of mild to moderate CAP.

1. JP Metlay et al. Diagnosis and treatment of adults with community-acquired pneumonia. An official clinical practice guideline of the American Thoracic Society and Infectious Diseases Society of America. Am J Respir Crit Care Med 2019; 200:e45.

2. N Horita et al. Adjunctive systemic corticosteroids for hospitalized community-acquired pneumonia: systematic review and meta-analysis 2015 update. Sci Rep 2015; 5:14061.

3. RA Siemieniuk et al. Corticosteroid therapy for patients hospitalized with community-acquired pneumonia: a systematic review and meta-analysis. Ann Intern Med 2015; 163:519.

4. S Jiang et al. Efficacy and safety of glucocorticoids in the treatment of severe community-acquired pneumonia: A meta-analysis. Medicine (Baltimore) 2019; 98:e16239.

5. M Briel et al. Corticosteroids in patients hospitalized with community-acquired pneumonia: systematic review and individual patient data metaanalysis. Clin Infect Dis 2018; 66:346.

6. LP Chen et al. Efficacy and safety of glucocorticoids in the treatment of community-acquired pneumonia: a meta-analysis of randomized controlled trials. World J Emerg Med 2015; 6:172.

7. M Confalonieri et al. Hydrocortisone infusion for severe community-acquired pneumonia: a preliminary randomized study. Am J Respir Crit Care Med 2005; 171:242.

8. RM Nafae et al. Adjuvant role of corticosteroids in the treatment of community-acquired pneumonia. Egypt J Chest Dis Tuberc 2013; 62:439.

9. MT James et al. CKD and risk of hospitalization and death with pneumonia. Am J Kidney Dis 2009; 54:24.

10. CA Blum et al. Adjunct prednisone therapy for patients with community-acquired pneumonia: a multicentre, double-blind, randomised, placebo-controlled trial. Lancet 2015; 385:1511.

11. A Torres et al. Effect of corticosteroids on treatment failure among hospitalized patients with severe community-acquired pneumonia and high inflammatory response: a randomized clinical trial. JAMA 2015; 313:677.

12. M Lloyd et al. Effectiveness of a bundled intervention including adjunctive corticosteroids on outcomes of hospitalized patients With community-acquired pneumonia: a stepped-wedge randomized clinical trial. JAMA 2019; 179:1052.

13. AK Waljee et al. Short-term use of oral corticosteroids and related harms among adults in the United States: population-based cohort study. BMJ 2017; 357:j1415.

14. C Rodrigo et al. Corticosteroids as adjunctive therapy in the treatment of influenza. Cochrane Database Syst Rev 2016; 3:CD010406.

15. A Rhodes et al. Surviving sepsis campaign: international guidelines for management of sepsis and septic shock: 2016. Intensive Care Med 2017; 43:304.

DRUGS FOR
Depression

Original publication date – February 2020 (revised September 2020)

Complete remission of symptoms is the goal of treatment for major depressive disorder; a partial response is associated with an increased risk of relapse. Improvement in symptoms can occur within the first two weeks of treatment with an antidepressant, but it may take 4-8 weeks to achieve a substantial benefit. Following successful treatment of a first major depressive episode, antidepressant treatment should be continued at the same dose for at least 4-9 months to consolidate recovery.[*] In patients with recurrent depressive episodes, long-term maintenance treatment can reduce the risk of relapse.[1]

A selective serotonin reuptake inhibitor (SSRI) is generally used for initial treatment of major depressive disorder. A serotonin-norepinephrine reuptake inhibitor (SNRI), bupropion (*Wellbutrin SR*, and others), and mirtazapine (*Remeron*, and generics) are reasonable alternatives.

SSRIs — There is no convincing evidence that any one SSRI is more effective than any other for treatment of major depressive disorder. Sertraline (*Zoloft*, and generics) or escitalopram (*Lexapro*, and generics) would be a reasonable choice for first-line treatment in adults. Fluoxetine (*Prozac*, and generics) is the only SSRI that is FDA-approved for treatment of major depressive disorder in children. Fluoxetine and escitalopram are both approved for treatment of major depressive disorder in adolescents.[2] SSRIs may not be effective for treatment of depression in patients with chronic nonpsychiatric disorders such as heart failure or chronic kidney disease.[3-5]

Adverse Effects – Restlessness, agitation, and sleep disturbances, particularly insomnia, can occur with use of SSRIs. Nausea, diarrhea, headache, dizziness, fatigue, and sexual dysfunction, which can include decreased libido, impaired arousal, delayed orgasm, or anorgasmia, can also occur.[6] SSRIs can cause hyponatremia, particularly in elderly patients. These drugs can increase the risk of bleeding by inhibiting serotonin uptake by platelets. QT interval prolongation has been reported with all SSRIs; the risk appears to be greatest with citalopram and escitalopram.[7,8] Some patients gain substantial amounts of weight with continued use of an SSRI, especially during the second and third years of treatment.[9] The long-term effects of SSRIs on the growth, personality development, and behavior of children remain to be established.

When SSRIs are stopped abruptly, discontinuation symptoms such as nervousness, anxiety, irritability, electric-shock sensations, bouts of tearfulness or crying, dizziness, lightheadedness, insomnia, confusion, trouble concentrating, nausea, and vomiting can occur; these effects are most severe with paroxetine (*Paxil*, and others), possibly because of its short half-life and potent serotonergic effects, and least likely to occur with fluoxetine because of its long half-life.

Drug Interactions – SSRIs vary in their effects on CYP isozymes and interact with many other drugs; some of these interactions are summarized in Table 2.

SNRIs — SNRIs are also considered first-line options for treatment of major depressive disorder. It is not clear that they offer any advantage in efficacy over SSRIs.

Adverse Effects – The adverse effects of SNRIs are similar to those of SSRIs, but can also include excessive sweating, constipation, tachycardia,

Summary: Drugs for Depression

▸ An SSRI, SNRI, bupropion, or mirtazapine can be used for first-line treatment of major depressive disorder, but most clinicians use an SSRI.

▸ All SSRIs appear to be similar in efficacy. Sertraline or escitalopram would be a reasonable choice for first-line treatment in adults. Fluoxetine would be a reasonable choice for treatment of children or adolescents.

▸ Bupropion can be used for treatment of major depressive disorder when anxiety is not a prominent symptom. It may be especially helpful in patients with impaired concentration, hypoactive sexual desire disorder, or antidepressant-induced sexual dysfunction.

▸ Mirtazapine may be useful in depressed patients with insomnia or marked weight loss.

▸ Tricyclic antidepressants and monoamine oxidase inhibitors are alternatives for patients with moderate to severe depression.

▸ When patients show little to no response to monotherapy, combining two antidepressants (but not two serotonergic drugs), such as bupropion and an SSRI, or adding another drug for augmentation, such as a second-generation antipsychotic, may be beneficial.

▸ Electroconvulsive therapy (ECT) has the highest rates of response and remission of any form of antidepressant therapy.

and urinary retention. Discontinuation symptoms can occur when these drugs are stopped abruptly, especially with venlafaxine (*Effexor XR*, and generics) and desvenlafaxine (*Pristiq*, and others) because of their short half-lives. SNRIs can cause dose-dependent increases in blood pressure; the risk is greatest with venlafaxine doses >150 mg/day. False-positive urine immunoassay screening tests for phencyclidine (PCP) and amphetamine have been reported in patients taking venlafaxine or desvenlafaxine.

Drug Interactions – SNRIs vary in their effects on CYP isozymes and interact with many other drugs; some of these interactions are summarized in Table 2.

BUPROPION — Bupropion, a norepinephrine and dopamine reuptake inhibitor, can be used as a first-line alternative to an SSRI or SNRI for treatment of major depressive disorder when anxiety is not a prominent

Table 1. Some Drugs for Depression

Drug	Some Available Formulations
Selective Serotonin Reuptake Inhibitors (SSRIs)	
Citalopram – generic	10, 20, 40 mg tabs; 2 mg/mL soln
Celexa (Allergan)	10, 20, 40 mg tabs
Escitalopram – generic	5, 10, 20 mg tabs; 1 mg/mL soln
Lexapro (Allergan)	5, 10, 20 mg tabs
Fluoxetine – generic	10, 20, 40 mg caps; 10, 20, 60 mg tabs; 4 mg/mL soln
Prozac (Lilly)	10, 20, 40 mg caps
delayed-release – generic	90 mg DR caps
Paroxetine HCl – generic	10, 20, 30, 40 mg tabs
Paxil (Apotex)	10, 20, 30, 40 mg tabs; 2 mg/mL susp
extended-release – generic	12.5, 25, 37.5 mg ER tabs
Paxil CR	
Paroxetine mesylate – *Pexeva* (Sebela)	20, 30, 40 mg tabs
Sertraline – generic	25, 50, 100 mg tabs; 20 mg/mL soln
Zoloft (Pfizer)	
Serotonin–Norepinephrine Reuptake Inhibitors (SNRIs)	
Desvenlafaxine succinate – generic	25, 50, 100 mg ER tabs
Pristiq (Pfizer)	
Desvenlafaxine – generic	50, 100 mg ER tabs
Duloxetine – generic	20, 30, 60 mg DR caps
Cymbalta (Lilly)	
Drizalma Sprinkle (Sun)	30, 40, 60 mg DR caps
Venlafaxine – generic	25, 37.5, 50, 75, 100 mg tabs
extended-release – generic	37.5, 75, 150 mg ER caps; 37.5, 75, 150, 225 mg ER tabs
Effexor XR (Pfizer)	37.5, 75, 150 mg ER caps

DR = delayed-release; ER = extended-release; ODT = orally disintegrating tablets; soln = solution; susp = suspension

1. Dosage adjustments may be needed for renal or hepatic impairment or for drug interactions. Lower initial dosages may be considered for elderly patients.
2. Approximate WAC for 30 days' treatment at the lowest usual adult dosage. WAC = wholesaler acquisition cost or manufacturer's published price to wholesalers; WAC represents a published catalogue or list price and may not represent an actual transactional price. Source: AnalySource® Monthly. February 5, 2020. Reprinted with permission by First Databank, Inc. All rights reserved. ©2020. www.fdbhealth.com/policies/drug-pricing-policy.

Initial Adult Dosage[1]	Usual Adult Dosage[1]	Cost[2]
20 mg once/day	20-40 mg once/day[3]	$2.40
		272.10
10 mg once/day	10-20 mg once/day[4]	4.80
		362.20
20 mg once/day	20-60 mg once/day	2.70[5]
		489.00
90 mg once/week	90 mg once/week	130.70
20 mg once/day	20-60 mg once/day	4.10
		202.50
12.5 mg once/day	25-75 mg once/day	83.90
		208.60
20 mg once/day	20-50 mg once/day	391.40
50 mg once/day	50-200 mg once/day	11.40
		350.90
50 mg once/day	50 mg once/day	161.00
		412.80
50 mg once/day	50 mg once/day	248.40
40-60 mg once/day	60-120 mg once/day	43.70
or divided bid	or divided bid	256.80
		175.50
37.5 mg once/day	75-375 mg/day	10.60
	divided bid or tid	
37.5-75 mg once/day	75-375 mg once/day	9.00[6]
		465.00

3. Maximum daily dose is 40 mg (20 mg in patients who are >60 years old, have hepatic impairment, are CYP2C19 poor metabolizers, or are taking a CYP2C19 inhibitor).
4. Maximum daily dose is 20 mg. The recommended dose for most elderly patients and those with hepatic impairment is 10 mg/day.
5. Cost of capsules. Cost for tablets is $20.10.
6. Cost of capsules. Cost for tablets is $115.30.

Continued on next page

Table 1. Some Drugs for Depression (continued)	
Drug	**Some Available Formulations**
Serotonin–Norepinephrine Reuptake Inhibitors (SNRIs) (continued)	
Levomilnacipran – *Fetzima* (Allergan)	20, 40, 80, 120 mg ER caps
Tricyclic Antidepressants (TCAs)[7]	
Amitriptyline – generic	10, 25, 50, 75, 100, 150 mg tabs
Amoxapine – generic	50, 100, 150 mg tabs
Desipramine – generic *Norpramin* (Validus)	10, 25, 50, 75, 100, 150 mg tabs 10, 25 mg tabs
Imipramine – generic	10, 25, 50 mg tabs
Imipramine pamoate – generic	75, 100, 125, 150 mg caps
Nortriptyline – generic	10, 25, 50, 75 mg caps; 2 mg/mL soln
Pamelor (Mallinckrodt)	10, 25, 50, 75 mg caps
Monoamine Oxidase Inhibitors (MAOIs)	
Isocarboxazid – *Marplan* (Validus)	10 mg tabs
Phenelzine – generic *Nardil* (Pfizer)	15 mg tabs
Selegiline – *Emsam* (Mylan)	6, 9, 12 mg/24 hr patches
Tranylcypromine – generic *Parnate* (Concordia)	10 mg tabs
Others	
Brexanolone – *Zulresso* (Sage Therapeutics)[8]	100 mg/20 mL single-use vials

DR = delayed-release; ER = extended-release; ODT = orally disintegrating tablets; soln = solution; susp = suspension
7. Narrow therapeutic index: serum concentrations should be monitored at steady state. Therapeutic serum concentrations are: amitriptyline 100-250 ng/mL; desipramine ≥125 ng/mL; imipramine ≥200 ng mL; nortriptyline 50-150 ng/mL.

Initial Adult Dosage[1]	Usual Adult Dosage[1]	Cost[2]
20 mg once/day x 2 days, then 40 mg once/day	40-120 mg once/day	$412.40
25-50 mg once/day or divided	100-300 mg once/day or divided	28.50
25-50 mg once/day, bid, or tid	200-300 mg/day divided bid or tid	88.10
25-50 mg once/day or divided	100-300 mg once/day or divided	82.90
		222.00
25-50 mg once/day or divided	100-300 mg once/day or divided	24.80
75 mg once/day	150 mg once/day	354.00
25 mg once/day	50-200 mg once/day or divided	29.40
		1226.00
10 mg bid	30-60 mg/day divided	446.10
15 mg tid	45-90 mg/day divided	58.50
		144.60
6 mg/24 hr	6, 9, 12 mg/24 hr	1756.80
10 mg once/day	20-30 mg bid	324.00
		883.50
See footnote 9	See footnote 9	37,250.00[10]

8. FDA-approved only for treatment of postpartum depression.
9. Administered as a continuous IV infusion over 60 hours at varying rates. At 0-4 and 56-60 hrs: 30 mcg/kg/hr; 4-24 and 52-56 hrs: 60 mcg/kg/hr; 24-52 hrs: 90 mcg/kg/hr. If the 90 mcg/kg/hr infusion is not tolerated, the dose can be reduced to 60 mcg/kg/hr.
10. Cost of 5 vials.

Continued on next page

Table 1. Some Drugs for Depression (continued)	
Drug	**Some Available Formulations**
Others (continued)	
Bupropion HCl – generic	75, 100 mg tabs
extended-release (12 hour) – generic	100, 150, 200 mg ER tabs
Wellbutrin SR (GSK)	
extended-release (24 hour) – generic	150, 300 mg ER tabs
Wellbutrin XL (Valeant)	
Forfivo XL (Almatica)	450 mg ER tabs
Bupropion hydrobromide – *Aplenzin*	174, 348, 522 mg ER tabs
(Valeant)	
Esketamine – *Spravato* (Janssen)	56, 84 mg kits
Mirtazapine – generic	7.5, 15, 30, 45 mg tabs
Remeron (Organon)	15, 30 mg tabs
orally disintegrating – generic	15, 30, 45 mg ODT
Remeron SolTab	
Nefazodone[13] – generic	50, 100, 150, 200, 250 mg tabs
Olanzapine/fluoxetine – generic	3/25, 6/25, 6/50, 12/25, 12/50 mg caps
Symbyax (Lilly)	3/25, 6/25, 6/50, 12/50 mg caps
Trazodone – generic	50, 100, 150, 300 mg tabs
Vilazodone – *Viibryd* (Allergan)	10, 20, 40 mg tabs
Vortioxetine – *Trintellix*	5, 10, 20 mg tabs
(Takeda/Lundbeck)	

DR = delayed-release; ER = extended-release; ODT = orally disintegrating tablets; soln = solution; susp = suspension
11. Initiate treatment with another bupropion formulation.
12. Administer 56 mg twice/week for weeks 1-4 and 56 mg or 84 mg once/week for weeks 5-8.

symptom. It is not sedating and has not been associated with weight gain, sexual dysfunction, or an increased risk of bleeding. Bupropion may be especially helpful in patients with impaired concentration, hypoactive sexual desire disorder, or antidepressant-induced sexual dysfunction.[10]

Adverse Effects – Bupropion can cause agitation, tremor, irritability, anxiety, insomnia, headache, nausea, anorexia, and hypertension. Dose-related seizures can occur.

Initial Adult Dosage[1]	Usual Adult Dosage[1]	Cost[2]
100 mg bid	100 mg tid	$63.00
150 mg once/day	150 mg bid	19.00
		445.30
150 mg once/day	300-450 mg once/day	78.30
		1940.20
See footnote 11	450 mg once/day	446.90
174 mg once/day	348 mg once/day	1962.40
56 mg intranasally x 1 dose[12]	56 or 84 mg intranasally q1 or 2 weeks[15]	1237.80
15 mg once/day at bedtime	15-45 mg once/day	6.00
		160.20
		53.00
		127.50
50 mg once/day	150-300 mg/day divided bid	78.50
6/25 mg once/day	6/25-12/50 mg once/day	321.80
		402.30[14]
75 mg bid	150-600 mg/day divided bid	36.10
10 mg once/day	20-40 mg once/day	285.90
10 mg once/day	10-20 mg once/day	383.70

13. Brand-name nefazodone (Serzone) was withdrawn from the market due to hepatotoxicity.
14. Wholesale cost according to the manufacturer.
15. The recommended dosage for treatment of patients with major depressive disorder (MDD) and acute suicidal ideation or behavior is 84 mg intranasally twice weekly for 4 weeks.

MIRTAZAPINE — Mirtazapine blocks presynaptic α_2-adrenergic receptors, increasing release of norepinephrine and serotonin. It may be particularly useful in patients with insomnia or marked weight loss. Mirtazapine may also be helpful in patients who experience significant nausea with SSRIs, SNRIs, or bupropion.

Adverse Effects – Mirtazapine can cause sedation, weight gain, dizziness, dry mouth, and constipation. Neutropenic fevers have occurred rarely.

Concurrent use with other serotonergic drugs can increase the risk of serotonin syndrome.

SECOND-LINE TREATMENT — When patients show little to no response to an adequate trial of an SSRI (4-8 weeks), many clinicians switch to another SSRI, an SNRI, or an antidepressant from a different class. Combining two antidepressants (but not two serotonergic drugs) from different classes, such as bupropion and an SSRI, or adding another drug for augmentation are additional alternatives.[1,11,12]

OTHER DRUGS — **Trazodone** is seldom used as monotherapy, but is commonly used in low doses at bedtime as an adjunct to an SSRI or SRNI in patients with insomnia. It can cause sedation, dizziness, nervousness, orthostatic hypotension, cardiovascular adverse effects, and priapism. **Nefazodone**, which is structurally similar to trazodone, has been withdrawn from the market in some countries because of severe hepatotoxicity.

Vilazodone *(Viibryd)*, which inhibits reuptake of serotonin and acts as a 5-HT_{1A} receptor partial agonist, is FDA-approved for treatment of major depressive disorder. There is no acceptable evidence for claims that it acts more rapidly than SSRIs.[13] Vilazodone has an adverse effect profile similar to that of SSRIs.

Vortioxetine *(Trintellix)*, which inhibits reuptake of serotonin and acts as a 5-HT_{1A} receptor agonist and 5-HT_3 receptor antagonist, is FDA-approved for treatment of major depressive disorder.[14] Vortioxetine has an adverse effect profile similar to that of SSRIs, but with less insomnia and more nausea and vomiting.

Tricyclic antidepressants (TCAs) and **monoamine oxidase inhibitors** (MAOIs) remain valuable alternatives for treatment of moderate to severe depression, despite concerns about their safety. **TCAs** have a narrow therapeutic index; serum concentrations should be monitored (see footnote 7 in Table 1). TCAs can cause anticholinergic adverse effects (urinary retention, constipation, dry mouth, blurred vision), orthostatic hypotension, weight gain, sedation, and sexual dysfunction. They can also cause QT interval prolongation[8] and cardiac conduction delays, and when taken in overdose, arrhythmias and death. TCAs must be used with caution in patients with ischemic heart disease and are generally not recommended for those with prolonged QRS or QTc intervals.

MAOIs are contraindicated for use with SSRIs, SNRIs, and other serotonergic, noradrenergic, and dopaminergic drugs, and their use requires strict adherence to a low tyramine diet to avoid life-threatening serotonin syndrome or hypertensive crisis. These interactions have not been reported with transdermal selegiline *(Emsam)* doses of 6 mg/day, but they can occur with higher doses.[15] The enzyme-inhibiting effects of MAOIs can persist for up to 2 weeks after the drug is stopped (during which time other serotonergic drugs are contraindicated). Adverse effects of MAOIs include sleep disturbances, orthostatic hypotension, sexual dysfunction, and weight gain.

A single IV infusion of the anesthetic agent **ketamine**, which can have dissociative effects, was effective for treatment of depression in several trials, but it is not approved by the FDA for such use.[16] Ketamine has been abused for its hallucinogenic effects for many years; it is classified as a schedule III controlled substance.

Esketamine *(Spravato)*, the S-enantiomer of ketamine, is FDA-approved for intranasal use in addition to an oral antidepressant in patients with treatment-resistant depression and has been more effective than placebo in inducing remission in such patients.[17,18] It has also recently been approved for treatment of depressive symptoms in adults with major depressive disorder (MDD) and acute suicidal ideation or behavior. Esketamine may temporarily improve scores on tests for depression, but there is no acceptable evidence that the drug reduces suicidal ideation or behavior compared to placebo.[51] It is administered under the direct supervision of a healthcare professional and is only available through a REMS program. Because of the risks of sedation and dissociation, patients must be monitored during and for at least 2 hours after administration of the drug. Esketamine is classified as a schedule III controlled substance.

Table 2. Some SSRI and SNRI Drug Interactions

Drug	CYP Properties/Effects
Selective Serotonin Reuptake Inhibitors (SSRIs)	
SSRI Class	Serotonergic effect
	QT interval prolongation
	Possible antiplatelet effect
Citalopram	Metabolized by 2C19[3] and 3A4
Escitalopram	Metabolized by 2C19[3] and 3A4
Fluoxetine[5]	Strong inhibitor of 2D6
	Moderate inhibitor of 2C19
	Metabolized by 2D6[3] and 2C9
Paroxetine	Strong inhibitor of 2D6
	Metabolized by 2D6
Sertraline[7]	Moderate inhibitor of 2D6
	Metabolized by 2C9, 2C19, 2D6, and 3A4
Serotonin-Norepinephrine Reuptake Inhibitors (SNRIs)	
SNRI Class	Serotonergic effect
	Possible antiplatelet effect
Desvenlafaxine	Weak inhibitor of 2D6
Duloxetine	Metabolized by 1A2[3] and 2D6
	Moderate inhibitor of 2D6
	Hepatic effects

1. Use of serotonergic drugs and monoamine oxidase inhibitors (MAOIs) concurrently or within 2 weeks of each other (3 weeks after vortioxetine and 5-6 weeks after fluoxetine) increases the risk of serotonin syndrome and is contraindicated.
2. QT interval prolongation has been reported with all SSRIs; the risk appears to be greatest with citalopram and escitalopram.
3. Primary pathway.
4. Inhibitors and inducers of CYP enzymes and P-glycoprotein. Med Lett Drugs Ther 2019 November 6 (epub). Available at medicalletter.org/downloads/CYP_PGP_Tables.pdf.

Comments

- ▶ Use of an SSRI with other serotonergic drugs may increase the risk of serotonin syndrome[1]
- ▶ Use of an SSRI with other QT-interval prolonging drugs could result in additive effects on the QT interval and an increased risk of torsades de pointes[2]
- ▶ Use of an SSRI with an antiplatelet or anticoagulant drug may increase the risk of bleeding

- ▶ Maximum dose of 20 mg/day in 2C19 poor metabolizers or with inhibitors of 2C19[4]

- ▶ Dosage adjustments may be needed with 2C19 inhibitors[4]

- ▶ May decrease efficacy of drugs that require 2D6 for activation and may increase concentrations of 2D6 substrates[6]
- ▶ May increase serum concentrations of phenytoin
- ▶ Strong 2D6 or 2C9 inhibitors can increase fluoxetine serum concentrations[4]

- ▶ May decrease efficacy of drugs that require 2D6 for activation and may increase concentrations of 2D6 substrates[6]
- ▶ Lower doses of paroxetine may be needed with 2D6 inhibitors[4]

- ▶ May increase concentrations of 2D6 substrates[6]
- ▶ Strong inducers of CYP enzymes may reduce sertraline serum concentrations[4]

- ▶ Use of an SNRI with other serotonergic drugs may increase the risk of serotonin syndrome[1]
- ▶ Use of an SNRI with an antiplatelet or anticoagulant drug may increase the risk of bleeding

- ▶ Reduce dose of 2D6 substrates by up to one-half if administered with 400 mg of desvenlafaxine[6]

- ▶ Avoid strong inhibitors of 1A2[4]
- ▶ 2D6 inhibitors can increase duloxetine concentrations[4]
- ▶ May increase concentrations of 2D6 substrates[6]
- ▶ Increased risk of hepatoxicity with heavy alcohol intake

5. Long half-life is a problem when interactions occur.
6. Tamoxifen, codeine, hydrocodone, and tramadol require 2D6 for conversion to their active metabolites. Drugs that are 2D6 substrates include tricyclic anti-depressants, aripiprazole, brexpiprazole, metoprolol, and propranolol.
7. Oral solution contains alcohol and may interact with disulfiram.

Continued on next page

Table 2. Some SSRI and SNRI Drug Interactions (continued)	
Drug	**CYP Properties/Effects**
Serotonin-Norepinephrine Reuptake Inhibitors (SNRIs) (continued)	
Levomilnacipran[8]	Metabolized by 3A4[3]
Venlafaxine	Metabolized by 2D6[3] and 3A4 QT interval prolongation

8. Alcohol increases release of the drug from extended-release capsules and should be avoided.

AUGMENTATION — Augmentation with a second-generation **antipsychotic drug** has been effective, but it can cause weight gain, metabolic adverse effects, and akathisia.[19-21] **Aripiprazole** (*Abilify*, and generics), **brexpiprazole** *(Rexulti)*,[22] and extended-release **quetiapine** (*Seroquel XR*, and generics) are FDA-approved for adjunctive treatment of major depressive disorder. A fixed-dose combination of **olanzapine and fluoxetine** (*Symbyax*, and generics) is FDA-approved for treatment-resistant depression.

Augmentation with low doses of **lithium** has been effective in some patients. When anxiety persists despite effective treatment of depression, augmentation with the anti-anxiety agent **buspirone** *(Buspar*, and generics) may be modestly helpful.[23]

WARNINGS — Suicidality – All FDA-approved antidepressants have a boxed warning in their labels regarding an increased risk of suicidal thinking and behavior in children, adolescents, and young adults. An FDA analysis of placebo-controlled trials found that antidepressant use increased suicidal thinking or behavior in patients ≤24 years old and decreased it in those ≥65 years old.[24] No increase in completed suicides has been documented among patients treated with antidepressants and in some studies, use of SSRIs was associated with less suicidal thinking and lower suicide rates in children and adolescents with depression.[25,26] All

Comments
▸ Dosage adjustment needed when administered with strong 3A4 inhibitors[4] (max 80 mg/day)
▸ Serum concentrations may be increased by 3A4 inhibitors[4] ▸ Use with other QT-interval prolonging drugs could result in additive effects on the QT interval and an increased risk of torsades de pointes

children, adolescents, and adults with depression should be monitored for suicidal ideation and behavior.

Mania – All antidepressants can induce mania, most often in patients with undetected or undiagnosed bipolar disorder. Patients should be screened for a personal or first-degree-relative history of mania, hypomania, or other evidence of bipolar disorder before starting antidepressant therapy, and those at risk should be followed closely in the first weeks to months of treatment.

Serotonin Syndrome – All serotonergic drugs can cause serotonin syndrome, a rare but potentially life-threatening condition characterized by altered mental status, fever, tachycardia, hypertension, agitation, tremor, myoclonus, hyperreflexia, ataxia, incoordination, diaphoresis, shivering, and GI symptoms.[27] Serotonin syndrome occurs rarely with SSRI monotherapy at recommended doses; it occurs most commonly as a result of interactions with other drugs. Serotonergic drugs and MAOIs should not be used concurrently or within 2 weeks of each other (3 weeks after vortioxetine and 5-6 weeks following fluoxetine). Some drugs with MAOI activity, such as the antimicrobial agent linezolid (*Zyvox*, and generics), and some that may not be recognized as serotonergic, such as dextromethorphan, tramadol (*Ultram*, and generics), triptans, methadone, and St. John's wort, can cause serotonin syndrome when taken concurrently with an SSRI or SNRI.[28] Use of opioids with serotonergic drugs can also cause serotonin syndrome.[29]

ALTERNATIVE PRODUCTS — L-methylfolate *(Deplin),* a prescription medical food, is marketed for patients who have major depressive disorder and suboptimal levels of L-methylfolate. Medical foods are regulated, but not reviewed or approved, by the FDA. Patients with reduced folate levels may be less likely to respond to antidepressant treatment and more likely to experience relapses. L-methylfolate is necessary for endogenous synthesis of serotonin, norepinephrine, and dopamine, and increased levels of these neurotransmitters have been associated with an improved response to antidepressant treatment.[30] There is no acceptable evidence, however, that L-methylfolate is effective for treatment of depression, whether or not the patient is folate-deficient.[31]

St. John's wort is available as a dietary supplement and is widely used for treatment of depression. The results of clinical trials supporting such use are mixed.[32] St. John's wort induces CY3A4, 2C19, and P-glycoprotein (P-gp) and interacts with many other drugs.[33] Its use with other serotonergic drugs or MAOIs can cause serotonin syndrome. As with all dietary supplements, the potency and purity of St. John's wort products can vary.

PREGNANCY — Nonpharmacologic treatment can be considered for mild depression, but untreated depression may be more harmful to the fetus than pharmacotherapy. Discontinuation of antidepressants during pregnancy may increase the risk of relapse. The potential for pregnancy should be considered when treating depression in women of child-bearing age.

SSRIs are the most frequently prescribed drugs for treatment of depression during pregnancy. The risk of congenital malformations after taking an SSRI during pregnancy appears to be very low, and no increase in perinatal mortality has been demonstrated.[34] An increased risk of cardiovascular and other malformations has been reported in infants born to mothers who took paroxetine in the first trimester.[35] Both untreated maternal depression and SSRI use during pregnancy have been associated with delayed fetal development, preterm birth, and low birth weight.[36] Taking an SSRI in the third trimester has been associated with a self-limited neonatal syndrome including motor, CNS, respiratory, and GI symptoms, treatment in a neonatal intensive care unit, and a possible risk of persistent pulmonary hypertension in the newborn.[37,38] The concentration of fluoxetine in breast milk is higher than that of most other SSRIs; its active metabolite has been detected in the serum of breastfed infants.

Studies of **SNRIs** during pregnancy are limited; increased risks of neonatal syndrome and perinatal complications have been reported with their use during pregnancy.[39]

The safety of **bupropion** during pregnancy has not been established. Studies of **mirtazapine** use during pregnancy are limited; no increased risk of congenital malformations has been observed.[40] **TCA** use during pregnancy has been associated with jitteriness and convulsions in newborns. Some clinicians do not recommend use of an **MAOI** during pregnancy because drug or food interactions could cause a hypertensive crisis. **Esketamine** is not recommended for use during pregnancy.

The long-term effects of maternal antidepressant use on child development are unclear. There is no convincing evidence that it increases the risk of attention-deficit/hyperactivity disorder (ADHD), autism spectrum disorder, or slow motor development in the offspring any more than depression itself.[41-43]

POSTPARTUM DEPRESSION — Up to 20% of women may experience postpartum depression (PPD) after childbirth. **SSRIs** are generally used for initial treatment of moderate to severe PPD, but data on their efficacy for this indication are mixed and maximal effects are only achieved after several weeks of treatment. **SNRIs** and **TCAs** have also been used, but data on their efficacy are limited.

Brexanolone *(Zulresso)*, a $GABA_A$ receptor modulator, is the first drug to be FDA-approved for treatment of PPD.[44,45] Administered as a continuous 60-hour IV infusion, it was modestly more effective than placebo in reducing post-infusion depressive symptom scores in women with moderate to severe PPD. The durability of the antidepressant effect of brexanolone is unclear and there is no evidence that it is more effective than SSRIs or other antidepressants for treatment of PPD. Brexanolone can cause excessive sedation and sudden loss of consciousness; it is only available through a REMS program. Continuous pulse oximetry is required during the infusion and the infusion should be stopped immediately and not restarted if hypoxia occurs. The cost of the drug alone for a single infusion is more than $35,000.[46] Brexanolone is classified as a schedule IV controlled substance.

NON-DRUG THERAPY — Electroconvulsive therapy (ECT) has the highest rates of response and remission of any form of antidepressant therapy (70-90%); it is highly effective for severe depression, depression with psychosis, bipolar depression, depressive catatonia, and treatment-resistant depression.[47] **Psychotherapy**, particularly **cognitive-behavioral therapy** (CBT) and **interpersonal therapy**, is effective for treatment of mild to moderately severe, nonpsychotic depression. **Transcranial magnetic stimulation** (TMS) and **vagus nerve stimulation** (VNS) are FDA-approved for treatment-resistant depression. TMS, unlike ECT, does not require anesthesia and does not appear to have cognitive adverse effects. In clinical trials, response and remission rates with TMS have been similar to those with antidepressants.[48] **Deep brain stimulation** (DBS) has been effective in a small number of patients with treatment-resistant depression, but it was not superior to sham treatment in clinical trials.[49,50]

1. American Psychiatric Association. Treating major depressive disorder: a quick reference guide. Based on practice guideline for the treatment of patients with major depressive disorder, third edition 2010. Available at http://bit.ly/2GTfF02. Accessed February 13, 2020.

2. A Cipriani et al. Comparative efficacy and tolerability of antidepressants for major depressive disorder in children and adolescents: a network meta-analysis. Lancet 2016; 388:881.

3. CE Angermann et al. Effect of escitalopram on all-cause mortality and hospitalization in patients with heart failure and depression: the MODD-HF randomized clinical trial. JAMA 2016; 315:2683.

4. SS Hedayati et al. Effect of sertraline on depressive symptoms in patients with chronic kidney disease without dialysis dependence: the CAST randomized clinical trial. JAMA 2017; 318:1876.

5. CP Walther et al. Treating depression in patients with advanced CKD: beyond the generalizability frontier. JAMA 2017; 318:1873.

6. MD Waldinger. Psychiatric disorders and sexual dysfunction. Handb Clin Neurol 2015; 130:469.

7. Citalopram, escitalopram and the QT interval. Med Lett Drugs Ther 2013; 55:59.

8. MC Funk et al. APA resource document. Resource document on QTc prolongation and psychotropic medications approved by the Joint Reference Committee, June 2018.

9. R Gafoor et al. Antidepressant utilisation and incidence of weight gain during 10 years' follow-up: population based cohort study. BMJ 2018; 361:k1951.

10. VM Pereira et al. Bupropion in the depression-related sexual dysfunction: a systematic review. CNS Neurol Disord Drug Targets 2014; 13:1079.

11. KR Connolly and ME Thase. If at first you don't succeed: a review of the evidence for antidepressant augmentation, combination and switching strategies. Drugs 2011; 71:43.

12. MH Trivedi et al. Medication augmentation after the failure of SSRIs for depression. N Engl J Med 2006; 354:1243.

13. Vilazodone (Viibryd) – a new antidepressant. Med Lett Drugs Ther 2011; 53:53.

14. Vortioxetine (Trintellix) for depression. Med Lett Drugs Ther 2013; 55:93.

15. Transdermal selegiline (Emsam). Med Lett Drugs Ther 2006; 48:41.

16. C Caddy et al. Ketamine and other glutamate receptor modulators for depression in adults. Cochrane Database Syst Rev 2015; 9:CD011612.

17. K Bozymski et al. Esketamine: A novel option for treatment-resistant depression. Ann Pharmacother 2019 Dec 4 (epub).

18. Esketamine nasal spray (Spravato) for treatment-resistant depression. Med Lett Drugs Ther 2019; 61:54.

19. Adjunctive antipsychotics for major depression. Med Lett Drugs Ther 2011; 53:74.

20. BM Wright et al. Augmentation with atypical antipsychotics for depression: a review of evidence-based support from the medical literature. Pharmacotherapy 2013; 33:344.

21. M Hobart et al. A long-term, open-label study to evaluate the safety and tolerability of brexpiprazole as adjunctive therapy in adults with major depressive disorder. J Clin Psychopharmacol 2019; 39:203.

22. Brexpiprazole (Rexulti) for schizophrenia and depression. Med Lett Drugs Ther 2015; 57:116.

23. MB Stein and J Sareen. Clinical practice. Generalized anxiety disorder. N Engl J Med 2015; 373:2059.

24. M Fornaro et al. The FDA "Black Box" warning on antidepressant suicide risk in young adults: more harm than benefits? Front Psychiatry 2019; 10:294.

25. J March et al. Fluoxetine, cognitive-behavioral therapy, and their combination for adolescents with depression: Treatment for Adolescents with Depression Study (TADS) randomized controlled trial. JAMA 2004; 292:807.

26. RD Gibbons et al. The relationship between antidepressant prescription rates and rate of early adolescent suicide. Am J Psychiatry 2006; 163:1898.

27. NA Buckley et al. Serotonin syndrome. BMJ 2014; 348:g1626.

28. EW Boyer and M Shannon. The serotonin syndrome. N Engl J Med 2005; 352:1112.

29. FDA. FDA Drug Safety Communication: FDA warns about several safety issues with opioid pain medicines; requires label changes. March 22, 2016. Available at: http://bit.ly/3bulrDo. Accessed February 13, 2020.

30. R Jain et al. Good, better, best: clinical scenarios for the use of L-methylfolate in patients with MDD. CNS Spectr 2019 Dec 13 (epub).

31. L-Methylfolate (Deplin) for depression and schizophrenia. Med Lett Drugs Ther 2010; 52:31.

32. RC Shelton. St. John's wort (Hypercum perforatum) in major depression. J Clin Psychiatry 2009; 70 (suppl 5):23.

33. Inhibitors and inducers of CYP enzymes and P-glycoprotein. Med Lett Drugs Ther 2019 November 6 (epub). Available at: medicalletter.org/downloads/CYP_PGP_Tables.pdf.

34. O Stephansson et al. Selective serotonin reuptake inhibitors during pregnancy and risk of stillbirth and infant mortality. JAMA 2013; 309:48.

35. A Bérard et al. Paroxetine use during pregnancy and perinatal outcomes including types of cardiac malformations in Quebec and France: a short communication. Curr Drug Saf 2012; 7:207.

36. H Malm et al. Pregnancy complications following prenatal exposure to SSRIs or maternal psychiatric disorders: results from population-based national register data. Am J Psychiatry 2015; 172:1224.

37. S Gentile. On categorizing gestational, birth, and neonatal complications following late pregnancy exposure to antidepressants: the prenatal antidepressant exposure syndrome. CNS Spectr 2010; 15:167.

38. CD Chambers et al. Selective serotonin-reuptake inhibitors and risk of persistent pulmonary hypertension of the newborn. N Engl J Med 2006; 354:579.

39. C Bellantuono et al. The safety of serotonin-noradrenaline reuptake inhibitors (SNRIs) in pregnancy and breastfeeding: a comprehensive review. Hum Psychopharmacol 2015; 30:143.

40. U Winterfeld et al. Pregnancy outcome following maternal exposure to mirtazapine: a multicenter, prospective study. J Clin Psychopharmacol 2015; 35:250.

41. LH Pedersen. The safety of antidepressant in pregnancy: maternal antidepressants are implicated in ADHD, but so is maternal depression. BMJ 2017; 357:j2544.

42. K Grove et al. Prenatal antidepressant exposure and child motor development: a meta-analysis. Pediatrics 2018; 142:e20180356.

43. T Boukhris et al. Antidepressant use during pregnancy and the risk of autism spectrum disorder in children. JAMA Pediatr 2016; 170:117.

44. Brexanolone (Zulresso) for postpartum depression. Med Lett Drugs Ther 2019; 61:68.

45. JG Powell et al. Brexanolone (Zulresso): finally, an FDA-approved treatment for postpartum depression. Ann Pharmacother 2020; 54:157.

46. Approximate WAC. WAC = wholesaler acquisition cost or manufacturer's published price to wholesalers; WAC represents a published catalogue or list price and may not represent an actual transactional price. Source: AnalySource® Monthly. February 5, 2020. Reprinted with permission by First Databank, Inc. All rights reserved. ©2020. www.fdbhealth.com/drug-pricing-policy.

47. PE Holtzheimer and HS Mayberg. Neuromodulation for treatment-resistant depression. F1000 Med Rep 2012; 4:22.
48. Health Quality Ontario. Repetitive transcranial magnetic stimulation for treatment-resistant depression: a systematic review and meta-analysis of randomized controlled trials. Ont Health Technol Assess Ser 2016; 16:1.
49. IO Bergfeld. Deep brain stimulation of the ventral anterior limb of the internal capsule for treatment-resistant depression: a randomized clinical trial. JAMA Psychiatry 2016; 73:456.
50. DD Dougherty. A randomized sham-controlled trial of deep brain stimulation of the ventral capsule/ventral striatum for chronic treatment-resistant depression. Biol Psychiatry 2015; 78:240.
51 A new indication for esketamine nasal spray (Spravato). Med Lett Drugs Ther 2020; 62:151.

Drugs Past Their Expiration Date

Original publication date – July 2020

Healthcare providers are often asked if drugs can be used past their expiration date. Because of legal restrictions and liability concerns, manufacturers do not sanction such use and usually do not comment on the safety or effectiveness of their products beyond the date on the label. Since our last article on this subject,[1] more data have become available.

SAFETY — There are no published reports of human toxicity due to ingestion, injection, or topical application of a currently available drug formulation after its expiration date. Renal tubular damage has been reported with use of degraded tetracycline in a formulation that is no longer manufactured.[2]

THE EXPIRATION DATE — The manufacturer's expiration date is based on the stability of the drug in the original sealed container. The date does not necessarily mean that the drug was found to be unstable after a longer period; it only means that real-time data or extrapolations from accelerated degradation studies indicate that the drug is expected to be stable on that date if stored in the closed container under recommended conditions. Most drug products have a labeled shelf life of 1-5 years, but in some cases (e.g., ophthalmic products), the expiration date on the original container no longer applies once it is opened.

STABILITY — Data from the US Department of Defense/FDA Shelf Life Extension Program, which tests the stability of drug products past their expiration date, have shown that 2650 of 3005 lots (88%) of 122 different products stored in their unopened original containers were able to have their shelf lives extended by an average of 66 months past the labeled expiration date.[3] Potassium iodide, which has been extensively stockpiled for use in a radiation emergency, has shown no significant degradation over many years.[4] A 2020 report from the US Department of Health and Human Services advised that it would be reasonable if necessary to use the antiviral products *Tamiflu* (oseltamivir; 75-mg capsules) and *Relenza* (zanamivir inhalation powder) for up to 15 and 10 years, respectively, after their date of manufacture if the products were stored under labeled conditions.[5]

HEAT, HUMIDITY, AND LONG-TERM STORAGE — Storage in high heat and/or humidity can accelerate the degradation of some drug formulations, but in one study, captopril tablets, theophylline tablets, and cefoxitin sodium powder for injection, stored at 40°C and 75% relative humidity, remained stable for 1.5-9 years beyond their expiration dates.[6] In another study, theophylline tablets retained 90% of their labeled content 30 years past their expiration date.[7] A study of 8 products that had been stored in their unopened original containers for 28-40 years past their expiration dates found that 12 of 14 active ingredients had retained ≥90% of their original potency; aspirin retained <5% of its potency, and amphetamine <60%.[8]

LIQUID FORMULATIONS — Solutions and suspensions are generally less stable than solid dosage forms, but in one report, 4 outdated samples of atropine solution (three up to 12 years past expiration and one >50 years past the expiration date) were all found to contain significant amounts of the drug.[9] Drugs in solution that have become cloudy or discolored or show signs of precipitation should not be used. Suspensions are particularly susceptible to freezing. Limiting factors with ophthalmic drugs include evaporation of the solvent and a decreasing ability of preservatives to inhibit microbial growth.[10]

EPINEPHRINE — Epinephrine solutions, which can reverse the life-threatening effects of allergic reactions, may lose potency after the expiration date. In a study of 34 auto-injectors that had expired within the previous 90 months, the decrease in epinephrine content was proportional to the number of months past the expiration date.[11] Multiple studies of epinephrine auto-injectors (including *EpiPen*, *EpiPen Jr*, *Auvi-Q*, and the generic for *Adrenaclick*) have found pens up to 6 years past their expiration dates to contain ≥80% of the labeled dose,[12-14] but these studies were not designed to detect the potential conversion of epinephrine from the active L-enantiomer to the inactive D-enantiomer.[15,16] One study of >100 pens that were 1-11 years past their expiration date and had been exposed to wide temperature ranges while stored in EMS vehicles found that only 12.6-31.3% of the labeled dose remained.[17]

NALOXONE — Available as injectable solutions and nasal sprays for reversal of opioid overdose, naloxone is now widely distributed to first responders and family members of opioid users, who may retain these products beyond their expiration date. In a 2019 study of naloxone samples collected from EMS or law enforcement training supplies and returns that had expired between 1990 and 2018, most samples were found to contain more than 90% of their labeled content.[18]

CONCLUSION — When no suitable alternative is available, outdated drugs may be effective. How much potency they retain varies with the drug, the formulation, the lot, the preservatives (if any), and the storage conditions, especially heat and humidity. Many solid dosage formulations stored under reasonable conditions in their original unopened containers retain ≥90% of their potency for at least 5 years after the expiration date on the label, and sometimes much longer. Solutions and suspensions are generally less stable. There are no published reports of toxicity from degradation products of currently available drugs.

1. Drugs past their expiration date. Med Lett Drugs Ther 2015; 57:164.
2. GW Frimpter et al. Reversible "Faconi syndrome" caused by degraded tetracycline. JAMA 1963; 184:111.
3. RC Lyon et al. Stability profiles of drug products extended beyond labeled expiration dates. J Pharm Sci 2006; 95:1549.

4. US Department of Health and Human Services. Guidance for federal agencies and state and local governments: potassium iodide tablets shelf life extension. March 2004. Available at: www.fda.gov/media/72521/download. Accessed July 16, 2020.

5. US Department of Health and Human Services. State antiviral drug stockpile HHS update: February 11, 2020. Available at: www.fda.gov/media/135460/download. Accessed July 16, 2020.

6. G Stark et al. A study of the stability of some commercial solid dosage forms beyond their expiration dates. Pharm J 1997; 258:637.

7. R Regenthal et al. The pharmacologic stability of 35-year old theophylline. Hum Exp Toxicol 2002; 21:343.

8. L Cantrell et al. Stability of active ingredients in long-expired prescription medications. Arch Intern Med 2012; 172:1685.

9. JG Schier et al. Preparing for chemical terrorism: stability of injectable atropine sulfate. Acad Emerg Med 2004; 11:329.

10. GD Novack. Can I use those eyedrops after the expiration date? Ocul Surf 2015; 13:169.

11. FE Simons et al. Outdated EpiPen and EpiPen Jr autoinjectors: past their prime? J Allergy Clin Immunol 2000; 105:1025.

12. O Rachid et al. Epinephrine doses contained in outdated epinephrine auto-injectors collected in a Florida allergy practice. Ann Allergy Asthma Immunol 2015; 114:354.

13. FL Cantrell et al. Epinephrine concentrations in EpiPens after the expiration date. Ann Intern Med 2017; 166:918.

14. L Kassel et al. Epinephrine drug degradation in autoinjector products. J Allergy Clin Immunol Pract 2019; 7:2491.

15. J Lan et al. Evaluation of epinephrine's expiration date: a US Food and Drug Administration's perspective. J Allergy Clin Immunol Pract 2019; 7:2948.

16. L Hollein and U Holzgrabe. Ficts and facts of epinephrine and norepinephrine stability in injectable solutions. Int J Pharm 2012; 434:468.

17. A Stonemen et al. Stability of epinephrine in expired EpiPen products from EMS ambulances. AAPS 2014; W5370.

18. S Pruyn et al. Quality assessment of expired naloxone products from first-responders' supplies. Prehosp Emerg Care 2019; 23:647.

DRUGS FOR
Hypertension

Original publication date – May 2020

Drugs available for treatment of chronic hypertension and their dosages, adverse effects, and costs are listed in the tables that begin on page 116. Treatment of hypertensive urgencies and emergencies is not discussed here.

NONPHARMACOLOGIC INTERVENTIONS — Adoption of a heart-healthy diet such as the Dietary Approaches to Stop Hypertension (DASH) diet,[1] limiting intake of sodium (ideally <1500 mg/day)[2] and alcohol (≤2 drinks/day for men and ≤1 drink/day for women),[3] and participation in a structured exercise program[4,5] are recommended for all adults with elevated blood pressure. Weight loss is recommended for adults who are overweight.[6] Potassium supplementation (target intake 3500-5000 mg/day), preferably through diet, is recommended for patients whose potassium intake is not restricted because of chronic kidney disease or use of a drug that decreases potassium excretion.[7]

PHARMACOLOGIC THERAPY — The goal of antihypertensive drug therapy recommended by the American College of Cardiology and American Heart Association is a blood pressure of <130/80 mm Hg.[8] All patients with a systolic blood pressure of ≥140 mm Hg or a diastolic pressure of ≥90 mm Hg should be treated with one or more antihypertensive drugs. Starting treatment with two drugs from different classes is recommended when baseline blood pressure is ≥20/10 mm Hg above goal and

---

Summary: Drugs for Hypertension

▶ The goal of antihypertensive drug therapy is a blood pressure of <130/80 mm Hg.

▶ Beginning treatment with two antihypertensive drugs from different classes is recommended when baseline blood pressure is ≥20/10 mm Hg above goal and should be considered when baseline blood pressure is ≥140/90 mm Hg.

▶ A thiazide-like diuretic, a calcium channel blocker, an angiotensin-converting enzyme (ACE) inhibitor, or an angiotensin receptor blocker (ARB) is recommended as initial therapy in the general population of hypertensive patients.

▶ A thiazide-like diuretic or calcium channel blocker is recommended for initial treatment of black patients, except for those with chronic kidney disease or heart failure, who should receive an ACE inhibitor or an ARB.

▶ An ACE inhibitor or an ARB is recommended for initial treatment of hypertension in non-black patients with diabetes. In the absence of albuminuria, a thiazide-like diuretic or calcium channel blocker would also be a reasonable choice.

▶ Beta blockers are recommended as initial therapy only for patients with another indication for a beta blocker, such as myocardial infarction or heart failure.

▶ Many patients with hypertension, especially black patients, need >1 drug to control their blood pressure. If the first drug does not achieve blood pressure goals, adding a second drug with a different mechanism of action is generally more effective than increasing the dose of the first drug and often allows for use of lower, better tolerated doses of both drugs.

▶ If an ACE inhibitor or an ARB was used initially, it is reasonable to add a thiazide-like diuretic or calcium channel blocker. Two or more renin-angiotensin system inhibitors should not be used concurrently.

---

should be considered when baseline blood pressure is ≥140/90 mm Hg. Patients with a blood pressure of 130-139/80-89 mm Hg do not require pharmacologic therapy unless their estimated 10-year atherosclerotic cardiovascular disease (ASCVD) risk[9] is ≥10% or they have diabetes, chronic kidney disease, heart failure, ischemic heart disease, or peripheral vascular disease.

DIURETICS — Thiazide and **thiazide-like diuretics** are often used for initial treatment of hypertension. Most positive studies used the long-acting thiazide-like diuretics **chlorthalidone** or **indapamide** and found them to be superior to other antihypertensive drugs in preventing heart failure and at least as effective in reducing cardiovascular and renal risk.[10]

Table 1. Initial Monotherapy for Hypertension	
General Population	
Non-black	THZD, ACE inhibitor, ARB, or CCB
Black	THZD or CCB
Chronic Kidney Disease (CKD)	
Non-black	ACE inhibitor or ARB
Black	ACE inhibitor or ARB
Diabetes	
Non-black	ACE inhibitor or ARB[1]
Black	THZD or CCB[2]

ACE = angiotensin-converting enzyme; ARB = angiotensin receptor blocker; CCB = calcium channel blocker; THZD = thiazide or thiazide-like diuretic
1. In the absence of albuminuria, a THZD or a CCB would also be a reasonable choice.
2. Black patients with both diabetes and CKD should receive an ACE inhibitor or an ARB.

Chlorthalidone and indapamide have longer durations of action than **hydrochlorothiazide**, and in most studies, they have been more effective.[11] In one cohort study in 730,225 patients, however, chlorthalidone was not associated with significant cardiovascular benefits compared to hydrochlorothiazide, and patients taking it had a higher risk of hypokalemia and other renal and electrolyte abnormalities.[12] **Metolazone** may be effective in patients with renal impairment when other thiazide or thiazide-like diuretics are not, but outcomes data are lacking.

Loop diuretics such as **furosemide** may be more effective than thiazide or thiazide-like diuretics in patients with moderate or severe renal impairment. **Ethacrynic acid** can be used in patients with allergies to nonantibiotic sulfonamides (thiazide diuretics and loop diuretics other than ethacrynic acid contain sulfonamide moieties).[13]

Potassium-sparing diuretics such as **amiloride** and **triamterene** are generally used with other diuretics to prevent or correct hypokalemia. They can cause hyperkalemia, particularly in patients with renal impairment and in those taking angiotensin-converting enzyme (ACE) inhibitors, angiotensin-receptor blockers (ARBs), beta blockers, or aliskiren.

Table 2. Some Oral Diuretics

Drug	Some Formulations
Thiazide and Thiazide-Like	
Chlorthalidone – generic	25, 50 mg tabs
Chlorothiazide – generic	500 mg tabs
Diuril (Salix)	250 mg/5 mL susp
Hydrochlorothiazide – generic	12.5 mg caps; 12.5, 25, 50 mg tabs
Indapamide – generic	1.25, 2.5 mg tabs
Metolazone[4] – generic	2.5, 5, 10 mg tabs
Loop	
Bumetanide[4] – generic	0.5, 1, 2 mg tabs
Ethacrynic acid[4] – generic	25 mg tabs
Edecrin (Valeant)	
Furosemide – generic	20, 40, 80 mg tabs; 10 mg/mL, 40 mg/5 mL soln
Lasix (Validus)	20, 40, 80 mg tabs
Torsemide – generic	5, 10, 20, 100 mg tabs
Potassium-Sparing	
Amiloride – generic	5 mg tabs
Triamterene[4] – generic	50, 100 mg caps
Dyrenium (Concordia)	
Mineralocorticoid Receptor Antagonists	
Eplerenone – generic	25, 50 mg tabs
Inspra (Pfizer)	
Spironolactone – generic	25, 50, 100 mg tabs
Aldactone (Pfizer)	
CaroSpir (CMP)	25 mg/5 mL susp

1. PK Whelton et al. J Am Coll Cardiol 2018; 71:2199. Dosage adjustments may be needed for renal or hepatic impairment or for drug interactions.
2. Approximate WAC for 30 days' treatment at the lowest usual adult dosage using the smallest whole number of dosage units. WAC = wholesaler acquisition cost or manufacturer's published price to wholesalers; WAC represents a published catalogue or list price and may not represent an actual transactional price. Source: AnalySource® Monthly. May 5, 2020. Reprinted with permission by First Databank, Inc. All rights reserved. ©2020. www.fdbhealth.com/policies/drug-pricing-policy.

Usual Adult Dosage[1]	Cost[2]	Frequent or Severe Adverse Effects[3]
12.5-25 mg once/day	$43.20	Hypokalemia, hypomagnesemia,
500-1000 mg once/ day or divided bid	89.20 80.10	hyperglycemia, hyponatremia, hypercalcemia, hyperuricemia,
25-50 mg once/day	1.10	hypercholesterolemia, hypertriglyceridemia,
1.25-2.5 mg once/day	9.30	pancreatitis, rash and other allergic
2.5-5 mg once/day	65.90	reactions, photosensitivity reactions
0.5-2 mg divided bid	31.70	Hypokalemia, hyponatremia,
50-200 mg once/day or divided bid	1197.40 1345.50	hypomagnesemia, hyperglycemia, metabolic alkalosis, hyperuricemia, blood
20-80 mg divided bid	1.20 17.90	dyscrasias, rash, hypercholesterolemia, hypertriglyceridemia, dehydration,
5-10 mg once/day	8.60	circulatory collapse
5-10 mg once/day or divided bid	19.70	Hyperkalemia, GI disturbances, rash, headache
50-100 mg once/day or divided bid	277.30 331.60	Hyperkalemia, GI disturbances, nephrolithiasis
50-100 mg once/day or divided bid	104.10 285.60	Hyperkalemia, hyponatremia
25-100 mg once/day	13.90 111.80 616.50	Hyperkalemia, hyponatremia, mastodynia, gynecomastia, menstrual abnormalities, GI disturbances, rash, erectile dysfunction, hair loss

3. Class effects. Some adverse effects may not have been reported with every drug in the class. Antihypertensive drugs may also interact with other drugs.
4. Not FDA-approved for treatment of hypertension.

Table 3. Some Oral Renin-Angiotensin System Inhibitors*

Drug	Some Formulations
Angiotensin-Converting Enzyme (ACE) Inhibitors	
Benazepril – generic	5, 10, 20, 40 mg tabs
Lotensin (Validus)	10, 20, 40 mg tabs
Captopril – generic	12.5, 25, 50, 100 mg tabs
Enalapril – generic	2.5, 5, 10, 20 mg tabs
Vasotec (Valeant)	
Epaned (Azurity)	1 mg/mL soln
Fosinopril – generic	10, 20, 40 mg tabs
Lisinopril – generic	2.5, 5, 10, 20, 30, 40 mg tabs
Prinivil (Merck)	5, 10, 20 mg tabs
Zestril (Almatica)	40 mg tabs
Qbrelis (Azurity)	1 mg/mL soln
Moexipril – generic	7.5, 15 mg tabs
Perindopril – generic	2, 4, 8 mg tabs
Quinapril – generic	5, 10, 20, 40 mg tabs
Accupril (Pfizer)	
Ramipril – generic	1.25, 2.5, 5, 10 mg caps
Altace (Pfizer)	
Trandolapril – generic	1, 2, 4 mg tabs

*Dual blockade of the renin-angiotensin system (RAS) increases the risk of hypotension, hyperkalemia, and acute renal failure. Combined use of RAS inhibitors should generally be avoided.
1. PK Whelton et al. J Am Coll Cardiol 2018; 71:2199. Dosage adjustments may be needed for renal or hepatic impairment or for drug interactions.
2. Approximate WAC for 30 days' treatment at the lowest usual adult dosage using the smallest whole number of dosage units. WAC = wholesaler acquisition cost or manufacturer's published price to wholesalers; WAC represents a published catalogue or list price and may not represent an actual transactional price. Source: AnalySource® Monthly. May 5, 2020. Reprinted with permission by First Databank, Inc. All rights reserved. ©2020. www.fdbhealth.com/policies/drug-pricing-policy.

Usual Adult Dosage[1]	Cost[2]	Frequent or Severe Adverse Effects[3]
10-40 mg once/day or divided bid	$8.90 57.40	Cough, hypotension (particularly with diuretic use or volume depletion), rash, acute renal failure in patients with bilateral renal artery stenosis or stenosis of the artery to a solitary kidney, angioedema, hyperkalemia (particularly if also taking potassium supplements or potassium-sparing diuretics), mild to moderate loss of taste, hepatotoxicity, pancreatitis, blood dyscrasias and renal damage (particularly in patients with renal dysfunction)
25-150 mg divided bid or tid	98.00	
5-40 mg once/day or divided bid	14.10 482.10 492.00	
10-40 mg once/day	8.80	
10-40 mg once/day	1.80 46.80 381.60 988.00	
7.5-30 mg once/day or divided bid	27.10	
4-16 mg once/day	16.40	
10-80 mg once/day or divided bid	5.00 121.30	
2.5-20 mg once/day or divided bid	7.40 149.40	
1-4 mg once/day	14.00	

3. Class effects. Some adverse effects may not have been reported with every drug in the class. Antihypertensive drugs may also interact with other drugs.

Continued on next page

Table 3. Some Oral Renin-Angiotensin System Inhibitors* (continued)	
Drug	**Some Formulations**
Angiotensin Receptor Blockers (ARBs)	
Azilsartan − *Edarbi* (Arbor)	40, 80 mg tabs
Candesartan − generic *Atacand* (AstraZeneca)	4, 8, 16, 32 mg tabs
Eprosartan − generic	600 mg tabs
Irbesartan − generic *Avapro* (Sanofi)	75, 150, 300 mg tabs
Losartan − generic *Cozaar* (Merck)	25, 50, 100 mg tabs
Olmesartan − generic *Benicar* (Daiichi Sankyo)	5, 20, 40 mg tabs
Telmisartan − generic *Micardis* (Boehringer Ingelheim)	20, 40, 80 mg tabs
Valsartan − generic *Diovan* (Novartis)	40, 80, 160, 320 mg tabs
Direct Renin Inhibitor	
Aliskiren − generic *Tekturna* (Novartis)	150, 300 mg tabs

The **mineralocorticoid receptor antagonists spironolactone** and **eplerenone** are effective for adjunctive treatment of refractory hypertension.[14,15] When added to standard treatment in patients who have heart failure with reduced ejection fraction (HFrEF), they have decreased the risk of hospitalization and death.[16] Both drugs are potassium-sparing. Eplerenone is selective for the mineralocorticoid receptor; it is less likely than spironolactone to cause gynecomastia at high doses.

ACE INHIBITORS — Angiotensin-converting enzyme (ACE) inhibitors are effective for treatment of hypertension and are generally well tolerated, except for the common side effect of cough. They are less effective in black patients unless combined with a thiazide-like diuretic or a calcium channel blocker. ACE inhibitors have been shown to reduce

Usual Adult Dosage[1]	Cost[2]	Frequent or Severe Adverse Effects[3]
40-80 mg once/day	$181.00	Similar to ACE inhibitors, rarely cause
8-32 mg once/day	86.20	cough or angioedema, reversible sprue-like
	97.00	enteropathy with olmesartan
600 mg once/day	82.20	
150-300 mg once/day	10.70	
	170.70	
50-100 mg once/day	5.40	
or divided bid	78.30	
20-40 mg once/day	158.30	
	192.00	
20-80 mg once/day	105.20	
	188.50	
80-320 mg once/day	14.70	
	203.90	
150-300 mg once/day	176.80	Same as ARBs, plus GI adverse effects
	207.80	(e.g., diarrhea)

mortality in patients without heart failure or left ventricular dysfunction who are at high risk for cardiovascular events, prolong survival in patients with heart failure with reduced ejection fraction (HFrEF) and in those with left ventricular dysfunction after a myocardial infarction, and reduce proteinuria in patients with either diabetic or nondiabetic nephropathy. Angioedema, a rare but potentially fatal adverse effect of ACE inhibitors, is significantly more common in black patients. ACE inhibitors should not be used with ARBs or aliskiren.

ARBs — Angiotensin receptor blockers (ARBs) are as effective as ACE inhibitors in lowering blood pressure and appear to be at least equally reno- and cardioprotective and are much less likely to cause cough or angioedema. Like ACE inhibitors, they are less effective in black patients

Table 4. Some Oral Calcium Channel Blockers

Drug	Some Formulations
Dihydropyridines	
Amlodipine besylate[4] – generic *Norvasc* (Pfizer)	2.5, 5, 10 mg tabs
Amlodipine benzoate – *Katerzia* (Azurity)	1 mg/mL oral susp
Felodipine – generic	2.5, 5, 10 mg ER tabs
Isradipine – generic	2.5, 5 mg caps
Nicardipine – generic	20, 30 mg caps

Nifedipine ER[5] – generic
   Adalat CC (Almatica)
   Procardia XL (Pfizer)
	30, 60, 90 mg ER tabs

Nisoldipine – generic *Sular* (Shionogi)	8.5, 17, 20, 25.5, 30, 34, 40 mg ER tabs 8.5, 17, 34 mg ER tabs
Nondihydropyridines	

Diltiazem[5] – generic (extended-release)
   Cardizem LA (Valeant)
   Matzim LA (Teva)
	180, 240, 300, 360, 420 mg ER tabs[6]

generic (extended-release)
   Taztia XT (Actavis)
   Tiadylt ER (Zydus)
   Tiazac (Valeant)
	120, 180, 240, 300, 360 mg ER caps[7]

generic (continuous-delivery)
   Cardizem CD (Valeant)
   Cartia XT (Actavis)
	120, 180, 240, 300, 360 mg ER caps[8]

generic (degradable) *Dilt-XR* (Apotex)	120, 180, 240 mg ER degradable caps
Verapamil – generic	40, 80, 120 mg tabs
long-acting – generic *Calan SR* (Pfizer)	120, 180, 240 mg SR tabs
generic *Verelan* (Kremers Urban)	120, 180, 240, 360 mg SR caps
generic *Verelan PM* (Kremers Urban)	100, 200, 300 mg ER caps

ER = extended-release; SR = sustained-release
1. PK Whelton et al. J Am Coll Cardiol 2018; 71:2199. Dosage adjustments may be needed for renal or hepatic impairment or for drug interactions.
2. Approximate WAC for 30 days' treatment at the lowest usual adult dosage using the smallest whole number of dosage units. WAC = wholesaler acquisition cost or manufacturer's published price to wholesalers; WAC represents a published catalogue or list price and may not represent an actual transactional price. Source: AnalySource® Monthly. May 5, 2020. Reprinted with permission by First Databank, Inc. All rights reserved. ©2020. www.fdbhealth.com/policies/drug-pricing-policy.

Usual Adult Dosage[1]	Cost[2]	Frequent or Severe Adverse Effects[3]
2.5-10 mg once/day	$2.10	Dizziness, headache, peripheral
	155.80	edema (more common than with
2.5-10 mg once/day	248.50	nondihydropyridines, more common
2.5-10 mg once/day	27.10	in women), flushing, tachycardia, rash,
5-10 mg divided bid	70.60	gingival hyperplasia
60-120 mg divided bid	138.00	
30-90 mg once/day	28.00	
	50.30	
	155.20	
17-34 mg once/day	182.80	
	565.30	
120-360 mg once/day	80.00	Dizziness, headache, edema, constipation
	135.10	(especially with verapamil), AV block,
	80.00	bradycardia, heart failure, lupus-like rash
	27.90	with diltiazem
	37.90	
	18.70	
	91.60	
	39.00	
	1276.30	
	39.80	
	24.70	
	26.40	
40-120 mg tid	6.40	
120-360 mg once/day	32.20	
or divided bid	221.60	
120-360 mg once/day	51.60	
	227.00	
100-300 mg qPM	59.10	
	200.10	

3. Class effects. Some adverse effects may not have been reported with every drug in the class. Antihypertensive drugs may also interact with other drugs.
4. Amlodipine is also available in combination with atorvastatin (*Caduet*, and generics) and celecoxib (*Consensi*).
5. Immediate-release nifedipine is not recommended for treatment of hypertension.
6. *Cardizem LA* is also available in 120-mg ER tabs.
7. *Tiadylt ER* and *Tiazac* are also available in 420-mg ER caps.
8. *Cartia XT* is not available in 360-mg ER caps.

Table 5. Some Oral Beta-Adrenergic Blockers

Drug	Some Formulations
Atenolol[4] – generic	25, 50, 100 mg tabs
Tenormin (Almatica)	
Betaxolol[4] – generic	10, 20 mg tabs
Bisoprolol[4] – generic	5, 10 mg tabs
Metoprolol[4] – generic	25, 37.5, 50, 75, 100 mg tabs
Lopressor (Validus)	50, 100 mg tabs
extended-release – generic	25, 50, 100, 200 mg ER tabs
Toprol-XL (AstraZeneca)	
Kapspargo Sprinkle (Sun)	25, 50, 100, 200 mg ER caps[5]
Nadolol – generic	20, 40, 80 mg tabs
Corgard (US Worldmeds)	
Propranolol – generic	10, 20, 40, 60, 80 mg tabs; 20 mg/5 mL, 40 mg/5 mL oral soln
extended-release – generic	60, 80, 120, 160 mg ER caps
Inderal LA (Ari)	
Inderal XL (Mist)	80, 120 mg ER caps
InnoPran XL (Akrimax)	80, 120 mg ER caps
Timolol – generic	5, 10, 20 mg tabs
Beta-Adrenergic Blockers with Intrinsic Sympathomimetic Activity	
Acebutolol[4] – generic	200, 400 mg caps
Pindolol – generic	5, 10 mg tabs
Beta-Adrenergic Blockers with Alpha-Blocking Properties	
Carvedilol – generic	3.125, 6.25, 12.5, 25 mg tabs
Coreg (GSK)	
extended-release – generic	10, 20, 40, 80 mg ER caps
Coreg CR (GSK)	
Labetalol – generic	100, 200, 300 mg tabs

ER = extended-release
1. PK Whelton et al. J Am Coll Cardiol 2018; 71:2199. Dosage adjustments may be needed for renal or hepatic impairment or for drug interactions.
2. Approximate WAC for 30 days' treatment at the lowest usual adult dosage using the smallest whole number of dosage units. WAC = wholesaler acquisition cost or manufacturer's published price to wholesalers; WAC represents a published catalogue or list price and may not represent an actual transactional price. Source: AnalySource® Monthly. May 5, 2020. Reprinted with permission by First Databank, Inc. All rights reserved. ©2020. www.fdbhealth.com/policies/drug-pricing-policy.

Usual Adult Dosage[1]	Cost[2]	Frequent or Severe Adverse Effects[3]
50-100 mg divided bid	$2.50	Fatigue, depression, bradycardia,
	381.60	erectile dysfunction, decreased
10-20 mg once/day	21.20	exercise tolerance, heart failure,
5-10 mg once/day	24.80	worsening of peripheral arterial
100-200 mg divided bid	3.20	insufficiency, may aggravate allergic
	115.20	reactions, bronchospasm, may mask
50-200 mg once/day	23.00	symptoms of and delay recovery
	35.90	from hypoglycemia, Raynaud's
	46.50	phenomenon, insomnia, vivid dreams
40-120 mg once/day	95.60	or hallucinations, hypertriglyceridemia,
	147.20	decreased HDL cholesterol, increased
80-160 mg divided bid	25.40	incidence of diabetes, sudden
		withdrawal may lead to exacerbation
80-160 mg once/day	48.50	of angina and myocardial infarction or
	530.50	precipitate thyroid storm
80-160 mg once/day at hs	681.40	
80-160 mg once/day at hs	681.40	
20-60 mg divided bid	81.70	
200-800 mg divided bid	12.50	Similar to other beta-adrenergic blockers,
10-60 mg divided bid	40.80	but with less resting bradycardia and lipid
		changes; acebutolol has been associated
		with a positive antinuclear antibody test
		and occasional drug-induced lupus
12.5-50 mg divided bid	9.30	Similar to other beta-adrenergic
	274.10	blockers, but more orthostatic
20-80 mg once/day	205.50	hypotension; hepatotoxicity with
	275.30	labetalol
200-800 mg divided bid	22.00	

3. Class effects. Some adverse effects may not have been reported with every drug in the class. Antihypertensive drugs may also interact with other drugs.
4. Cardioselective.
5. Capsules can be opened and their contents sprinkled over soft food such as applesauce, pudding, or yogurt and consumed within 60 minutes.

Continued on next page

Table 5. Some Oral Beta-Adrenergic Blockers (continued)	
Drug	**Some Formulations**
Beta-Adrenergic Blocker with Nitric Oxide-Mediated Vasodilatory Activity	
Nebivolol[4] – *Bystolic*	2.5, 5, 10, 20 mg tabs

6. J Fongemie and E Felix-Getzik. Drugs 2015; 75:1349.

unless combined with a thiazide-like diuretic or a calcium channel blocker. ARBs should not be used with ACE inhibitors or aliskiren.

DIRECT RENIN INHIBITOR — Aliskiren is FDA-approved for use alone or in combination with other antihypertensive drugs for treatment of hypertension.[17] It has not been shown to have any advantage over an ACE inhibitor or an ARB. Aliskiren should not be used with an ACE inhibitor or an ARB.

CALCIUM CHANNEL BLOCKERS — The calcium channel blockers are structurally and functionally heterogeneous. They all cause vasodilation and decrease total peripheral resistance. The cardiac response to decreased vascular resistance is variable; some **dihydropyridines (felodipine, nicardipine**, and **nisoldipine**) cause an initial reflex tachycardia, but others (**isradipine, nifedipine**, and **amlodipine**) generally have a lesser effect on heart rate. The immediate-release formulation of nifedipine is not recommended for treatment of hypertension. The **nondihydropyridines verapamil** and **diltiazem** slow heart rate and can slow atrioventricular conduction; they should be used with caution in patients who are also taking a beta blocker.

In a large outcomes trial (ACCOMPLISH), the ACE inhibitor benazepril plus amlodipine was more effective in reducing adverse cardiovascular events than benazepril plus hydrochlorothiazide.[18]

BETA-ADRENERGIC BLOCKERS — A beta blocker may be an acceptable choice for treatment of hypertension in patients with another

Usual Adult Dosage[1]	Cost[2]	Frequent or Severe Adverse Effects[3]
5-40 mg once/day	$119.50	Similar to other beta-adrenergic blockers, but with less erectile dysfunction[6]

indication for a beta blocker, such as migraine headache prophylaxis, certain cardiac arrhythmias, angina pectoris, myocardial infarction, or heart failure, and possibly in younger patients (<60 years old) and in those with hyperkinetic circulation (palpitations, tachycardia, anxiety).[19] One meta-analysis of cardiovascular outcomes trials found that when beta blockers were used for treatment of hypertension, they were less effective in preventing cardiovascular events (especially stroke) than ACE inhibitors, ARBs, calcium channel blockers, and diuretics.[20] Like ACE inhibitors and ARBs, beta blockers are less effective in black patients.

Acebutolol and **pindolol** have intrinsic sympathomimetic activity (ISA). Beta blockers without ISA are preferred in patients with angina or a history of myocardial infarction. **Carvedilol** and **labetalol** block both beta- and alpha-adrenergic receptors. Compared with **metoprolol**, carvedilol may be less likely to interfere with glycemic control in patients with type 2 diabetes.[21] **Nebivolol** does not have alpha-blocking properties at clinically relevant doses, but it does have nitric oxide-mediated vasodilatory activity.[22,23]

ALPHA-ADRENERGIC BLOCKERS — **Doxazosin**, **prazosin**, and **terazosin** cause less tachycardia than direct vasodilators, but they are more likely to cause postural hypotension, especially after the first dose and in the elderly, and they can increase the risk of falling. Treatment of essential hypertension with doxazosin, compared to treatment with chlorthalidone, has been associated with an increased incidence of heart failure, stroke, and combined cardiovascular disease.[24] Alpha blockers provide symptomatic

Table 6. Some Oral Alpha-Adrenergic Blockers, Central Alpha-Adrenergic Agonists

Drug	Some Formulations
Alpha-Adrenergic Blockers	
Doxazosin – generic *Cardura* (Pfizer) extended-release – *Cardura XL*[4]	1, 2, 4, 8 mg tabs 4, 8 mg ER tabs
Prazosin – generic *Minipress* (Pfizer)	1, 2, 5 mg caps
Terazosin – generic	1, 2, 5, 10 mg caps
Central Alpha-Adrenergic Agonists	
Clonidine – generic *Catapres* (Boehringer Ingelheim)	0.1, 0.2, 0.3 mg tabs[5]
Guanfacine – generic	1, 2 mg tabs
Methyldopa – generic	250, 500 mg tabs
Direct Vasodilators	
Hydralazine – generic	10, 25, 50, 100 mg tabs
Minoxidil – generic	2.5, 10 mg tabs

ER = extended-release
1. PK Whelton et al. J Am Coll Cardiol 2018; 71:2199. Dosage adjustments may be needed for renal or hepatic impairment or for drug interactions.
2. Approximate WAC for 30 days' treatment at the lowest usual adult dosage using the smallest whole number of dosage units. WAC = wholesaler acquisition cost or manufacturer's published price to wholesalers; WAC represents a published catalogue or list price and may not represent an actual transactional price. Source: AnalySource® Monthly. May 5, 2020. Reprinted with permission by First Databank, Inc. All rights reserved. ©2020. www.fdbhealth.com/policies/drug-pricing-policy.

Direct Vasodilators

Usual Adult Dosage[1]	Cost[2]	Frequent or Severe Adverse Effects[3]
1-16 mg once/day	$19.30	Syncope with first dose (less likely with
	116.60	terazosin and doxazosin), dizziness
4-8 mg once/day	134.10	and vertigo, headache, palpitations,
2-20 mg divided	76.40	fluid retention, drowsiness, weakness,
bid or tid	260.70	anticholinergic effects, priapism,
1-20 mg once/day	4.50	thrombocytopenia, atrial fibrillation
or divided bid		
0.2-0.8 mg divided bid	3.20	CNS reactions (similar to methyldopa, but
	142.30	more sedation and dry mouth), bradycardia, heart block, rebound hypertension (less likely with patch), contact dermatitis from patch
1-2 mg once/day[6]	8.10	Similar to clonidine, but milder
500-1000 mg divided bid	10.50	Sedation, fatigue, depression, dry mouth, orthostatic hypotension, bradycardia, heart block, autoimmune disorders (including colitis, hepatitis), hepatic necrosis, Coombs-positive lupus-like syndrome, thrombocytopenia, red cell aplasia, erectile dysfunction, hemolytic anemia
100-200 mg divided bid or tid	11.50	Tachycardia, aggravation of angina, headache, dizziness, fluid retention, nasal congestion, lupus-like syndrome, hepatitis
5-100 mg once/day or divided bid or tid	15.20	Tachycardia, aggravation of angina, marked fluid retention (coadministration of a loop diuretic is required), pericardial effusion, hirsutism

3. Class effects. Some adverse effects may not have been reported with every drug in the class. Antihypertensive drugs may also interact with other drugs.
4. Not FDA-approved for treatment of hypertension.
5. Clonidine is also available as extended-release transdermal patches (*Catapres TTS*, and generics). The usual dosage is one patch (0.1, 0.2, or 0.3 mg/24 hrs) applied once every 7 days.
6. The first dose is 1 mg at bedtime; 1-mg doses of the drug provide all or most of its antihypertensive effect and are generally well tolerated.

Table 7. Some Oral Combination Products

Drug	Some Formulations	Cost[1]
ACE Inhibitors and Diuretics		
Benazepril/HCTZ	5/6.25, 10/12.5, 20/12.5,	
generic	20/25 mg tabs[2]	$38.20
Lotensin HCT (Validus)		60.90
Captopril/HCTZ	25/15, 25/25, 50/15,	
generic	50/25 mg tabs	29.20
Enalapril/HCTZ		
generic	5/12.5, 10/25 mg tabs	16.20
Vaseretic (Valeant)	10/25 mg tabs	391.10
Fosinopril/HCTZ	10/12.5, 20/12.5 mg tabs	
generic		43.20
Lisinopril/HCTZ	10/12.5, 20/12.5, 20/25 mg	
generic	tabs	5.20
Zestoretic (Almatica)		381.60
Quinapril/HCTZ	10/12.5, 20/12.5, 20/25 mg	
generic	tabs	27.10
Accuretic (Pfizer)		117.90
ARBs and Diuretics		
Azilsartan/chlorthalidone	40/12.5, 40/25 mg tabs	
Edarbyclor (Arbor)		170.90
Candesartan/HCTZ	16/12.5, 32/12.5, 32/25 mg	
generic	tabs	105.80
Atacand HCT (AstraZeneca)		131.30
Irbesartan/HCTZ	150/12.5, 300/12.5 mg tabs	
generic		22.30
Avalide (Sanofi)		206.50
Losartan/HCTZ	50/12.5, 100/12.5,	
generic	100/25 mg tabs	7.00
Hyzaar (Merck)		116.10
Olmesartan/HCTZ	20/12.5, 40/12.5, 40/25 mg	
generic	tabs	158.30
Benicar HCT (Daiichi Sankyo)		192.00

ACE = angiotensin-converting enzyme; ARB = angiotensin receptor blocker; ER = extended-release; HCTZ = hydrochlorothiazide
1. Approximate WAC for 30 days' treatment at the lowest usual adult dosage using the smallest whole number of dosage units. WAC = wholesaler acquisition cost or manufacturer's published price to wholesalers; WAC represents a published catalogue or list price and may not represent an actual transactional price. Source: AnalySource® Monthly. May 5, 2020. Reprinted with permission by First Databank, Inc. All rights reserved. ©2020. www.fdbhealth.com/policies/drug-pricing-policy.
2. *Lotensin HCT* is not available in 5/6.25-mg tabs.

Continued on next page

Table 7. Some Oral Combination Products (continued)

Drug	Some Formulations	Cost[1]
ARBs and Diuretics (continued)		
Telmisartan/HCTZ	40/12.5, 80/12.5, 80/25 mg	
generic	tabs	$115.00
Micardis HCT		188.50
(Boehringer Ingelheim)		
Valsartan/HCTZ	80/12.5, 160/12.5, 160/25,	
generic	320/12.5, 320/25 mg tabs	30.90
Diovan HCT (Novartis)		229.30
Direct Renin Inhibitor and Diuretic		
Aliskiren/HCTZ	150/12.5, 150/25, 300/12.5,	
Tekturna HCT (Novartis)	300/25 mg tabs	165.10
Beta-Adrenergic Blockers and Diuretics		
Atenolol/chlorthalidone	50/25, 100/25 mg tabs	
generic		16.40
Tenoretic (Almatica)		450.00[3]
Bisoprolol/HCTZ	2.5/6.25, 5/6.25, 10/6.25 mg	
generic	tabs	12.10
Ziac (Teva)		170.40
Metoprolol succinate/HCTZ	25/12.5, 50/12.5,	
generic	100/12.5 mg ER tabs	1249.50
Dutoprol (Concordia)		184.00
Metoprolol tartrate/HCTZ	50/25, 100/25, 100/50 mg	
generic	tabs	27.20
Lopressor HCT (Validus)	50/25 mg tabs	62.10
Nadolol/bendroflumethiazide	80/5 mg tabs	
generic		111.80
Propranolol/HCTZ	40/25, 80/25 mg tabs	
generic		27.60
Beta-Adrenergic Blocker and ARB		
Nebivolol/valsartan	5/80 mg tabs	
Byvalson (Allergan)		109.60
Calcium Channel Blockers and ACE Inhibitors		
Amlodipine/benazepril	2.5/10, 5/10, 5/20, 5/40	
generic	10/20, 10/40 mg caps[4]	27.30
Lotrel (Novartis)		246.50

3. Cost for 100/25-mg tabs. The cost for thirty 50/25-mg tabs is 1080.00.
4. *Lotrel* is not available in 2.5/10-mg caps.

Continued on next page

Table 7. Some Oral Combination Products (continued)		
Drug	**Some Formulations**	**Cost[1]**
Calcium Channel Blockers and ACE Inhibitors (continued)		
Amlodipine/perindopril	2.5/3.5, 5/7, 10/14 mg tabs	
Prestalia (Symplmed)		$156.20
Verapamil ER/trandolapril	180/2, 240/1, 240/2,	
generic	240/4 mg tabs[5]	127.00
Tarka (AbbVie)		167.90
Calcium Channel Blockers and ARBs		
Amlodipine/telmisartan	5/40, 5/80, 10/40, 10/80 mg	
generic	tabs	126.30
Twynsta (Boehringer Ingelheim)		202.80
Amlodipine/valsartan	5/160, 5/320, 10/160,	
generic	10/320 mg tabs	44.10
Exforge (Novartis)		230.20
Amlodipine/olmesartan	5/20, 5/40, 10/20, 10/40 mg	
generic	tabs	88.50
Azor (Daiichi Sankyo)		249.40
Calcium Channel Blocker and Direct Renin Inhibitor		
Amlodipine/aliskiren	5/150, 10/150, 5/300,	
Tekamlo (Novartis)	10/300 mg tabs	131.00
Diuretic Combinations		
HCTZ/spironolactone	25/25 mg tabs	
generic		36.00
Aldactazide (Pfizer)	25/25, 50/50 mg tabs	65.30
HCTZ/triamterene	25/37.5, 50/75 mg tabs,	
generic	25/37.5, 25/50 mg caps	9.00
Dyazide (GSK)	25/37.5 mg caps	62.60
Maxzide (Mylan)	25/37.5, 50/75 mg tabs	45.50
HCTZ/amiloride	50/5 mg tabs	
generic		12.20
Central Alpha-Adrenergic Agonist and Diuretic		
Methyldopa/HCTZ	250/15, 250/25 mg tabs	
generic		44.00

ACE = angiotensin-converting enzyme; ARB = angiotensin receptor blocker; ER = extended-release; HCTZ = hydrochlorothiazide
5. *Tarka* is not available in 240/1-mg tabs.

Continued on next page

Table 7. Some Oral Combination Products (continued)		
Drug	Some Formulations	Cost[1]
ARB/Calcium Channel Blocker/Diuretic Combinations		
Valsartan/amlodipine/HCTZ generic	160/5/12.5, 160/5/25, 160/10/12.5, 160/10/25,	$111.70
Exforge HCT (Novartis)	320/10/25 mg tabs	230.20
Olmesartan/amlodipine/HCTZ generic	20/5/12.5, 40/5/12.5, 40/5/25, 40/10/12.5,	122.60
Tribenzor (Daiichi Sankyo)	40/10/25 mg tabs	239.40

relief from benign prostatic hyperplasia (BPH) in men, but they may cause stress incontinence in women. It is not clear that they have any place in the treatment of hypertension, except as second-line agents in men with BPH.

CENTRAL ALPHA-ADRENERGIC AGONISTS — **Clonidine**, **guanfacine**, and **methyldopa** decrease sympathetic outflow, but they do not inhibit reflex responses as completely as sympatholytic drugs that act peripherally. Once-daily guanfacine may be a reasonable add-on for treatment of refractory hypertension. Central alpha-adrenergic agonists can cause sedation, dry mouth, and erectile dysfunction.

DIRECT VASODILATORS — Direct vasodilators frequently produce reflex tachycardia (especially early in treatment) and rarely cause orthostatic hypotension. They should generally be given with a beta blocker or a centrally acting drug to minimize the reflex increase in heart rate and cardiac output, and with a diuretic to manage sodium and fluid retention. The maintenance dose of **hydralazine** should be limited to 200 mg/day to decrease the possibility of a lupus-like reaction. **Minoxidil**, a potent drug that rarely fails to lower blood pressure, should be reserved for severe hypertension refractory to other drugs. It may cause hirsutism and tachycardia, and can also cause severe fluid retention; concomitant use of a loop diuretic is necessary.

PREGNANCY — Drugs affecting the renin-angiotensin system (**ACE inhibitors**, **ARBs**, and **aliskiren**) have been associated with serious fetal toxicity, including renal and cardiac abnormalities and death; they are contraindicated for use during pregnancy.

Methyldopa has a long history of safe use in pregnancy, but the high doses often required to adequately lower blood pressure can cause significant sedation.

Calcium channel blockers are generally considered safe for use during pregnancy.

A review of 13 population-based studies found that use of **beta blockers** in the first trimester did not result in an overall increase in congenital malformations, but analyses of organ-specific malformations found that their use was associated with increased rates of cleft lip/palate and cardiovascular and neural tube defects.[25]

Thiazide and **thiazide-like diuretics** should not be initiated during pregnancy because the volume depletion caused by these drugs in their first weeks of use may reduce uteroplacental perfusion. Women already taking a thiazide or thiazide-like diuretic who become pregnant can generally continue taking it.

1. FM Sacks et al. Effects on blood pressure of reduced dietary sodium and the Dietary Approaches to Stop Hypertension (DASH) diet. N Engl J Med 2001; 344:3.
2. D Mozaffarian et al. Global sodium consumption and death from cardiovascular causes. N Engl J Med 2014; 371:624.
3. M Roerecke et al. The effect of a reduction in alcohol consumption on blood pressure: a systematic review and meta-analysis. Lancet Public Health 2017; 2:e108.
4. SP Whelton et al. Effect of aerobic exercise on blood pressure: a meta-analysis of randomized, controlled trials. Ann Intern Med 2002; 136:493.
5. JD Inder et al. Isometric exercise training for blood pressure management: a systematic review and meta-analysis to optimize benefit. Hypertens Res 2016; 39:88.
6. JE Neter et al. Influence of weight reduction on blood pressure: a meta-analysis of randomized controlled trials. Hypertension 2003; 42:878.
7. PK Whelton et al. Effects of oral potassium on blood pressure. Meta-analysis of randomized controlled clinical trials. JAMA 1997; 277:1624.
8. PK Whelton et al. 2017 ACC/AHA/AAPA/ABC/ACPM/AGS/APhA/ASH/ASPC/NMA/ PCNA guideline for the prevention, detection, evaluation, and management of high blood

pressure in adults: executive summary: a report of the American College of Cardiology/ American Heart Association Task Force on Clinical Practice Guidelines. J Am Coll Cardiol 2018; 71:2199.

9. American College of Cardiology. ASCVD risk estimator plus. Available at: http://tools. acc.org/ASCVD-Risk-Estimator-Plus. Accessed May 7, 2020.

10. JT Wright Jr et al. ALLHAT findings revisited in the context of subsequent analyses, other trials, and meta-analyses. Arch Intern Med 2009; 169:832.

11. GC Roush et al. Diuretics: a review and update. J Cardiovasc Pharmacol Ther 2014; 19:5.

12. G Hripcsak et al. Comparison of cardiovascular and safety outcomes of chlorthalidone vs hydrochlorothiazide to treat hypertension. JAMA Intern Med 2020; 180:542.

13. Sulfonamide cross-reactivity. Med Lett Drugs Ther 2019; 61:44.

14. DA Calhoun et al. Refractory hypertension: determination of prevalence, risk factors, and comorbidities in a large, population-based cohort. Hypertension 2014; 63:451.

15. DA Calhoun and WB White. Effectiveness of the selective aldosterone blocker, eplerenone, in patients with resistant hypertension. J Am Soc Hypertens 2008; 2:462.

16. Drugs for chronic heart failure. Med Lett Drugs Ther 2019; 61:49.

17. Aliskiren (Tekturna) for hypertension. Med Lett Drugs Ther 2007; 49:29.

18. K Jamerson et al. Benazepril plus amlodipine or hydrochlorothiazide for hypertension in high-risk patients. N Engl J Med 2008; 359:2417.

19. WH Frishman and E Saunders. ß-adrenergic blockers. J Clin Hypertens (Greenwich) 2011; 13:649.

20. CS Wiysonge et al. Beta-blockers for hypertension. Cochrane Database Syst Rev 2017; 1:CD002003.

21. GL Bakris et al. Metabolic effects of carvedilol vs metoprolol in patients with type 2 diabetes mellitus and hypertension: a randomized controlled trial. JAMA 2004; 292:2227.

22. Nebivolol (Bystolic) for hypertension. Med Lett Drugs Ther 2008; 50:17.

23. J Fongemie and E Felix-Getzik. A review of nebivolol pharmacology and clinical evidence. Drugs 2015; 75:1349.

24. ALLHAT Collaborative Research Group. Major cardiovascular events in hypertensive patients randomized to doxazosin vs chlorthalidone: the antihypertensive and lipid-lowering treatment to prevent heart attack trial (ALLHAT). JAMA 2000; 283:1967.

25. MY Yakoob et al. The risk of congenital malformations associated with exposure to β-blockers early in pregnancy: a meta-analysis. Hypertension 2013; 62:375.

DRUGS FOR
Irritable Bowel Syndrome

Original publication date – March 2020

Irritable bowel syndrome (IBS) is a common disorder characterized by recurrent abdominal pain and altered bowel habits, often accompanied by bloating.[1,2] IBS is classified according to the predominant bowel symptom as IBS with constipation (IBS-C), IBS with diarrhea (IBS-D), mixed type (IBS-M), or unclassified (IBS-U). Alterations in the microbiome, stress responses, sensory and motor function of the gut, and host genetic factors may be contributing factors. Since the exact cause of IBS is unknown, the goal of treatment is symptom control.

NONPHARMACOLOGIC AND ALTERNATIVE TREATMENTS

DIET — Many patients with IBS have symptoms associated with meals or specific foods. A diet low in fermentable oligosaccharides, disaccharides, monosaccharides, and polyols **(FODMAPs)** may reduce IBS symptoms.[3] FODMAPs are poorly absorbed, rapidly fermented, short-chain carbohydrates that can increase gas production and induce osmosis in the intestinal lumen, causing bloating and abdominal pain; some common sources of FODMAPs are apples, stone fruits, onions, garlic, milk, yogurt, wheat, high-fructose corn syrup, and artificial sweeteners.[4] Data relating to the efficacy of **gluten** avoidance in patients with IBS are conflicting.[5,6] A meta-analysis examining two randomized, controlled trials of a gluten-free diet and seven randomized, controlled trials of a

---

Summary: Drugs for IBS

- ▶ Symptoms often respond to dietary and lifestyle changes; a low-FODMAP diet and exercise may be helpful.
- ▶ Probiotics may improve abdominal pain, bloating, and flatulence, but optimal probiotic species, strains, and dosages remain to be established.
- ▶ Peppermint oil or other antispasmodics can be used for abdominal pain or post-prandial symptoms.
- ▶ Antidepressants (TCAs or SSRIs) can reduce abdominal pain in patients with moderate to severe symptoms.
- ▶ Psychological interventions such as cognitive behavioral therapy have been effective in reducing symptoms.

Drugs for IBS with Constipation (IBS-C)

- ▶ Soluble fiber can improve symptoms.
- ▶ Polyethylene glycol (*Miralax*, and others) can increase the frequency of bowel movements, but may not improve global IBS symptoms.
- ▶ Lubiprostone *(Amitiza)*, linaclotide *(Linzess)*, plecanatide *(Trulance)*, or tenapanor *(Ibsrela)* may be modestly effective in patients who have not responded to fiber and polyethylene glycol.

Drugs for IBS with Diarrhea (IBS-D)

- ▶ Antidiarrheals such as loperamide are effective in reducing stool frequency, but do not improve global IBS symptoms.
- ▶ Rifaximin *(Xifaxan)* for 14 days is effective in relieving symptoms, but symptoms often recur and repeat courses of treatment may be required.
- ▶ Eluxadoline *(Viberzi)* has produced a modest improvement in symptoms. The risk of pancreatitis limits its use.
- ▶ Alosetron *(Lotronex)* should be reserved for women with severe, chronic IBS-D unresponsive to other drugs.

---

low-FODMAP diet found a non-significant trend towards global IBS symptom improvement with gluten avoidance and a significant improvement in symptoms with a low FODMAP diet.[7]

EXERCISE — The most recent American College of Gastroenterology (ACG) guidelines recommend including exercise in the management of IBS.[1] Several studies have suggested that physical activity, including yoga, may improve global IBS symptoms (pain, discomfort, bloating).[8-11]

FIBER — A meta-analysis of 15 studies found that soluble (psyllium), but not insoluble (bran), fiber decreased IBS symptoms.[12] Fiber can increase gas production and cause bloating, flatulence, and abdominal discomfort; slow titration of the dose can minimize these effects.

PEPPERMINT OIL — Peppermint oil, which has anti-spasmodic properties due to blockade of calcium channels, is available over the counter (OTC). In two randomized, controlled trials, peppermint oil was superior to placebo in decreasing abdominal pain, abdominal discomfort, and IBS symptom severity.[13,14] Peppermint oil is generally well tolerated; the most common adverse effect is heartburn.

PROBIOTICS — Changes in intestinal flora may contribute to IBS symptoms through a variety of mechanisms, including differential fermentation and gas production, changes in gut mucosa, and alterations in gut permeability.[15] A meta-analysis of 24 randomized, controlled trials in patients with IBS found that probiotics improved abdominal pain, bloating, and flatulence.[16] The optimal species, strains, and dosages of probiotics for treatment of IBS have not been established. Probiotics can cause gas, diarrhea, and bloating; these effects are usually mild and transient.[17]

PSYCHOLOGICAL INTERVENTIONS — Several psychological interventions, including cognitive behavioral therapy (CBT), relaxation training, and hypnotherapy, have been effective for management of IBS symptoms.[18] In a randomized, controlled trial, addition of telephone- or web-delivered CBT was effective in reducing IBS symptoms compared to usual treatment alone.[19]

DRUGS FOR ABDOMINAL PAIN OR DISCOMFORT

ANTISPASMODICS — Antispasmodics available by prescription such as **hyoscyamine** (*Levsin*, and others) and **dicyclomine** (*Bentyl*, and generics) induce intestinal smooth muscle relaxation through direct

Table 1. Some OTC Products for Irritable Bowel Syndrome (IBS)

Drugs[1]	Some Available Formulations
Soluble Fiber	
Psyllium – *Metamucil* (P&G)	5.8 g/teaspoon powder; 5.8 g packets; 1.8 g caps; 2 g wafers
Methylcellulose – *Citrucel* (GSK)	2 g/tablespoon powder; 500 mg caplets
Wheat dextrin – *Benefiber* (GSK)	4 g/teaspoon powder; 4, 6.2 g packets; chewable tabs
Calcium polycarbophil – *FiberCon* (Pfizer)	625 mg caplets
Antispasmodic	
Peppermint oil – generic *Pepogest* (Nature's Way) *IBgard*[11] (IM Health Sciences)	50 mg enteric-coated caps 0.2 mL enteric-coated caps 90 mg sustained-release caps
Osmotic Laxative	
Polyethylene glycol – *Miralax* (Bayer)	17 g/scoop powder; 17 g packets
Antidiarrheals	
Loperamide – *Imodium A-D* (Johnson & Johnson)	2 mg caplets; 1 mg/7.5 mL oral soln

OTC = over the counter; soln = solution
1. Individual retailers may have their own generic products.
2. Approximate cost at walgreens.com. Accessed March 11, 2020.
3. Should be taken with 8 ounces of water. Start with a single dose and increase gradually to improve tolerability.
4. Take at least 2 hours before or after taking other drugs.
5. For products available in powder formulations, the cost listed is for a *Metamucil* canister containing 114 teaspoons of powder, a *Citrucel* canister with 907 g of powder, a *Benefiber* canister with 500 g of powder, or a *Miralax* canister with 510 g of powder.
6. Should be taken with 4-8 ounces of water or other non-carbonated beverage or sprinkled on hot or cold soft food.

myorelaxant effects or anticholinergic mechanisms and may improve IBS symptoms.[20] Antispasmodics are often used as needed for acute attacks of abdominal pain, or before meals in patients with postprandial symptoms such as pain, gas, bloating, or fecal urgency.

Adverse Effects – High doses of **hyoscyamine** and **dicyclomine** can cause anticholinergic adverse effects including visual disturbances, confusion, dry mouth, urinary retention, palpitations, and constipation.

Usual Adult Dosage	Cost[2]
10-15 g/day in 2-3 divided doses[3,4]	$21.99[5]
2 g tid[3]	25.99[5]
8 g tid[6]	24.99[5]
3 tabs tid	
1250 mg once/day-qid[3]	21.99[7]
1-3 caps tid[8]	9.99[9]
1 cap tid[8]	28.98[10]
180 mg tid[12]	119.96[13]
17 g once/day-bid	24.99[5]
2 mg as needed (max 16 mg/day)	23.98[14]

7. Cost for 140 caplets.
8. Should be taken 30-60 minutes before meals.
9. Approximate cost for 90 capsules manufactured by Mason Natural.
10. Approximate cost for 2 packages containing 60 capsules each.
11. Enteric-coated sustained-release microsphere formulation marketed as a medical food.
12. Should be taken with water 30-90 minutes before or after food. The capsules should not be crushed or chewed. The capsule can be opened and the contents sprinkled on applesauce and ingested.
13. Approximate cost for 4 packages containing 48 capsules each.
14. Cost for 48 caplets.

Drug Interactions – Antispasmodics may affect the absorption of other drugs. Use with drugs that also have anticholinergic properties may result in additive effects.

ANTIDEPRESSANTS — Antidepressants can reduce abdominal pain and alter GI transit time. They are generally used in IBS when symptoms (particularly abdominal pain) are moderate to severe. A meta-analysis found that patients taking a **tricyclic antidepressant (TCA)** were more likely to experience symptom improvement than those taking placebo. Results of studies with **selective serotonin reuptake inhibitors (SSRIs)** have been more variable, but SSRIs have also been found to improve symptoms.[18] TCAs can cause constipation and may be particularly useful for patients with IBS-D. Conversely, SSRIs can cause diarrhea and may be helpful for patients with IBS-C.

Adverse Effects – TCAs can cause fatigue, dizziness, weight gain, sedation, and anticholinergic adverse effects including dry mouth, urinary retention, blurred vision, confusion, and constipation; they should be used with caution in patients with IBS-C. **SSRIs** can cause agitation, sleep disturbances, nausea, weight gain, sexual dysfunction, and diarrhea, and therefore should be used with caution in patients with IBS-D. All FDA-approved antidepressants have a boxed warning in their labels regarding an increased risk of suicidal thinking and behavior in children, adolescents, and young adults.

Drug Interactions – All **TCAs** are primarily metabolized by CYP2D6; concurrent use of drugs that inhibit CYP2D6 can increase serum concentrations of TCAs and possibly their toxicity.[21] SSRIs are metabolized by various CYP isozymes and they interact with many other drugs.[22] Concurrent use of SSRIs or TCAs with other drugs that prolong the QT interval could increase the risk of life-threatening arrhythmias such as torsades de pointes. Use of SSRIs with other serotonergic drugs could result in serotonin syndrome. Some drugs that may not be recognized as serotonergic, but could cause serotonin syndrome when taken with an SSRI include dextromethorphan, tramadol (*Ultram*, and others), triptans, methadone, and St. John's wort.

PREGABALIN — Pregabalin (*Lyrica*, and generics) is a calcium channel alpha-2-delta ligand that acts as a GABA analog and has both analgesic and anxiolytic effects. In one randomized, double-blind trial in 85 patients with IBS, 12 weeks of pregabalin treatment significantly reduced mean bowel symptom scale scores for pain or discomfort compared to placebo.[23]

Adverse Effects – Pregabalin can cause peripheral edema, dizziness, somnolence, weight gain, ataxia, dry mouth, blurred vision, and confusion. It is classified as a schedule V controlled substance because euphoria has been associated with its use.

DRUGS FOR IBS-C

OSMOTIC LAXATIVES — The OTC osmotic laxative **polyethylene glycol** (PEG; *Miralax*, and generics) can increase the frequency of bowel movements in patients with IBS-C, but there is no evidence that it improves overall symptoms or abdominal pain associated with IBS.[24] It is well tolerated and safe for long-term use.

CHLORIDE CHANNEL ACTIVATOR — **Lubiprostone** *(Amitiza)* is a prostaglandin derivative that activates GI chloride channels, stimulating intestinal fluid secretion.[25] It is FDA-approved for treatment of IBS-C in women ≥18 years old. In two 12-week, randomized, double-blind trials, lubiprostone provided greater relief of IBS symptoms than placebo; in a combined analysis, 18% of patients taking lubiprostone were considered overall responders compared to 10% of those taking placebo.[26] In a withdrawal trial, lubiprostone responders were re-randomized to continue lubiprostone or switch to placebo. After 4 weeks, lubiprostone was not more effective than placebo in maintaining a response (38% vs 40%).[27]

Adverse Effects – Nausea (8%) and diarrhea (7%) are the most common adverse effects of lubiprostone. Dyspnea has been reported rarely.

Drug Interactions – Methadone may reduce activation of chloride channels in the gut by lubiprostone.

GUANYLATE CYCLASE-C AGONISTS — **Linaclotide** *(Linzess)* and **plecanatide** *(Trulance)* are FDA-approved for treatment of IBS-C in adults.[28] They target guanylate cyclase-C receptors on the intestinal epithelium, resulting in increased cyclic guanosine monophosphate

Table 2. Some Drugs for Irritable Bowel Syndrome (IBS)

Drugs	Some Available Formulations
Drugs for Abdominal Pain or Discomfort	
Antispasmodics	
Dicyclomine[3] – generic	10 mg caps; 20 mg tabs; 10 mg/5 mL soln
Hyoscyamine[3] – generic	0.125 mg tabs; 0.125 mg ODT, SL tabs; 0.125 mg/5 mL elixir; 0.125 mg/mL soln
Anaspaz (Ascher)	0.125 mg ODT
Levsin (Meda)	0.125 mg tabs
Levsin-SL	0.125 mg SL tabs
extended-release – generic	0.375 mg ER tabs
Levbid (Meda)	
Selective Serotonin Reuptake Inhibitors (SSRIs)	
Citalopram[3] – generic	10, 20, 40 mg tabs; 40 mg ODT; 2 mg/mL soln
Celexa (Allergan)	10, 20, 40 mg tabs
Fluoxetine[3] – generic	10, 20, 40 mg caps; 10, 20, 60 mg tabs; 20 mg/5 mL soln
Prozac (Lilly)	10, 20, 40 mg caps
Paroxetine[3] – generic	10, 20, 30, 40 mg tabs
Paxil (Apotex)	10, 20, 30, 40 mg tabs; 10 mg/5 mL susp
extended-release – generic	12.5, 25, 37.5 mg ER tabs
Paxil CR	
Tricyclic Antidepressants (TCAs)	
Amitriptyline[3] – generic	10, 25, 50, 75, 100, 150 mg tabs
Desipramine[3] – generic	10, 25, 50, 75, 100, 150 mg tabs
Norpramin (Validus)	
Nortriptyline[3] – generic	10, 25, 50, 75 mg caps; 10 mg/5 mL soln
Pamelor (Mallinckrodt)	10, 25, 50, 75 mg caps
Other	
Pregabalin[3,5] – generic	25, 50, 75, 100, 150, 200, 225, 300 mg caps; 20 mg/mL soln
Lyrica (Pfizer)	

ER = extended-release; ODT = orally disintegrating tablets; soln = solution; SL = sublingual; susp = suspension
1. Dosage adjustments may be needed for renal or hepatic impairment or for drug interactions.
2. Approximate WAC for 30 days' treatment at the lowest usual adult dosage. WAC = wholesaler acquisition cost or manufacturer's published price to wholesalers; WAC represents a published catalogue or list price and may not represent an actual transactional price. Source: AnalySource® Monthly. March 5, 2020. Reprinted with permission by First Databank, Inc. All rights reserved. ©2020. www.fdbhealth.com/policies/drug-pricing-policy.

Usual Adult Dosage[1]	Cost[2]
20-40 mg qid prn	$33.60
0.125-0.25 mg tid-qid prn	41.80
	22.30
	215.20
	215.20
0.375-0.75 mg bid	61.80
	244.90
20-40 mg once/day[4]	5.60
	283.80
20 mg once/day	5.40
	489.00
10-20 mg once/day	8.50
	184.80
12.5-37.5 mg once/day	129.70
	199.90
10-75 mg once/day	4.10
10-125 mg once/day or divided bid	27.50
	46.40
10-125 mg once/day or divided bid	6.70
	1178.70
75-225 mg bid[6]	30.80
	516.00

3. Not FDA-approved for treatment of IBS.
4. Maximum dose is 40 mg (20 mg in patients who are >60 years old, have hepatic impairment, are CYP2C19 poor metabolizers, or are taking a 2C19 inhibitor).
5. Classified as a schedule V controlled substance.
6. In one trial in patients with IBS, pregabalin was given in escalating doses of 75 mg twice daily for 3 days, then 150 mg twice daily for 3 days, followed by the maintenance dose of 225 mg twice daily for 10 weeks. The drug was then tapered in week 12 (150 mg twice daily for 3 days, then 75 mg twice daily for 3 days).

Continued on next page

Table 2. Some Drugs for Irritable Bowel Syndrome (IBS) (continued)

Drugs	Some Available Formulations
Drugs for IBS with Constipation (IBS-C)	
Chloride Channel Activator	
Lubiprostone[7,8] – *Amitiza* (Takeda)	8, 24 mcg caps
Guanylate Cyclase-C Agonists	
Linaclotide[8] – *Linzess* (Allergan/Ironwood)	72, 145, 290 mcg caps
Plecanatide[8] – *Trulance* (Salix)	3 mg tabs
Sodium-Hydrogen Exchanger 3 (NHE3) Inhibitor	
Tenapanor[12] – *Ibsrela* (Ardelyx)	50 mg tabs
5-HT$_4$ Agonists	
Tegaserod[14] – *Zelnorm* (Alfasigma)	6 mg tabs
Drugs for IBS with Diarrhea (IBS-D)	
Antibiotic	
Rifaximin – *Xifaxan* (Salix)	200, 550 mg tabs
Bile Acid Sequestrants	
Cholestyramine[3] – generic *Questran* (Par)	4 g packets; 4 g/scoop
Colesevelam[3] – generic *Welchol* (Daiichi Sankyo)	625 mg tabs; 3.75 g packets
Colestipol[3] – generic *Colestid* (Pfizer)	1 g tabs; 5 g packets; 5 g/scoop 1 g tabs; 5, 7.5 g packets; 5 g/scoop
Mu-Opioid Receptor Agonist/Delta-Opioid Receptor Antagonist	
Eluxadoline[20] – *Viberzi* (Allergan)	75, 100 mg tabs

ER = extended-release; ODT = orally disintegrating tablets; soln = solution; SL = sublingual; susp = suspension; N.A. = cost not yet available

7. FDA-approved for treatment of IBS-C in women ≥18 years old.
8. Also FDA-approved for treatment of chronic idiopathic constipation (CIC).
9. Should be taken with meals and ≥8 ounces of water to minimize nausea. The recommended dosage should be reduced to 8 mcg once/day in IBS-C patients with severe hepatic impairment.
10. Should be taken in the morning 30 minutes before eating. The capsules should not be crushed or chewed. The capsules can be opened and the contents sprinkled on applesauce or dispersed in water and ingested.
11. Tablets can be crushed and mixed with room temperature applesauce or dissolved in water and ingested.
12. FDA-approved, but not yet available.
13. Should be taken immediately before breakfast or the first meal of the day and immediately before dinner.

Usual Adult Dosage[1]	Cost[2]
8 mcg bid[9]	$371.10
290 mcg once/day[10]	445.00
3 mg once/day[11]	436.50
50 mg bid[13]	N.A.
6 mg bid[15]	408.50
550 mg tid x 14 days[16]	1788.80[17]
4-16 g/day in divided doses	61.50[18] 170.60[18]
3.75 g once/day or in divided doses	455.40 657.00
5-30 g/day in divided doses[19]	94.30[18] 201.50[18]
100 mg bid[21]	1317.40

14. FDA-approved only for use in women with IBS-C who are <65 years of age and do not have a history of MI, angina, stroke, or transient ischemic attack.
15. Should be taken at least 30 minutes before eating.
16. Can be repeated up to 2 times if symptoms recur.
17. Cost for 14 days' treatment.
18. Cost for a 30-day supply of packets.
19. Effective dosage for IBS-D not well studied.
20. Classified as a schedule IV controlled substance.
21. Should be taken with food. The recommended dosage is 75 mg bid for patients who cannot tolerate the usual dosage, are receiving concomitant treatment with an OATP1B1 inhibitor, or have mild to moderate hepatic impairment.

Continued on next page

Table 2. Some Drugs for Irritable Bowel Syndrome (IBS) (continued)	
Drugs	**Some Available Formulations**
Drugs for IBS with Diarrhea (IBS-D) (continued)	
5-HT Modulators	
Alosetron[22] – generic *Lotronex* (Sebela)	0.5, 1 mg tabs

Ondansetron[3] – generic
  Zofran (Novartis)
	4, 8, 24 mg tabs; 4, 8 mg ODT;
	  4 mg/5 mL soln

ER = extended-release; ODT = orally disintegrating tablets; soln = solution; SL = sublingual; susp = suspension
22. Alosetron is FDA-approved only for use in women with severe IBS-D who have chronic symptoms (≥6 months) and no abnormalities of the GI tract, and whose IBS has not responded adequately to conventional treatment. Prescribers are expected to complete training as part of a Risk Evaluation and Mitigation Strategy (REMS) program.

(cGMP), which in turn activates the cystic fibrosis transmembrane conductance regulator ion channel, increasing luminal intestinal secretions and accelerating intestinal transit.

In a randomized, double-blind, 12-week trial in 800 patients with IBS-C, significantly more patients taking **linaclotide** achieved the primary endpoint for response (a ≥30% decrease in abdominal pain and at least 1 more spontaneous bowel movement from baseline for at least 6 of 12 weeks) compared to those taking placebo (34% vs 21%).[29] A 26-week trial produced similar results.[30]

In two randomized, double-blind, 12-week trials in a total of 2189 patients with IBS-C, more patients taking **plecanatide** achieved the primary endpoint for response compared to those taking placebo (30% vs 18% and 22% vs 14%); these differences are statistically significant.[31]

Adverse Effects – The most common adverse effects of guanylate cyclase-C agonists are diarrhea (20% with linaclotide and 4% with plecanatide), abdominal pain, flatulence, and abdominal distention. The labeling of both drugs includes a boxed warning against use in patients

Usual Adult Dosage[1]	Cost[2]
0.5-1 mg bid[23]	$837.40
	2132.70
4 mg once/day[24]	16.00
	697.70

23. If IBS is not controlled after 4 weeks of treatment with alosetron 1 mg bid, the drug should be discontinued.
24. K Garsed et al. Gut 2014; 63:1617.

<18 years old because of a risk of serious dehydration. Linaclotide and plecanatide are contraindicated for use in children <6 years old and in patients with intestinal obstruction.

NHE3 INHIBITOR — **Tenapanor** *(Ibsrela)* is the first sodium-hydrogen exchanger 3 (NHE3) inhibitor to be FDA-approved for the treatment of IBS-C in adults. It inhibits sodium absorption in the small intestine and colon, resulting in increased fluid secretion and acceleration of intestinal transit time. In two randomized, double-blind trials, the primary endpoint for response (a ≥30% decrease in abdominal pain at least 1 more spontaneous bowel movement from baseline for at least 6 of 12 weeks) was achieved in significantly more patients taking tenapanor compared to those taking placebo (27% vs 19% and 37% vs 24%).[32,33]

Adverse Effects – Diarrhea (16%), flatulence, and abdominal distention (3% each) have been the most common adverse effects of tenapanor. As with linaclotide and plecanatide, the labeling of tenapanor includes a boxed warning about the risk of serious dehydration in children. The drug is contraindicated for use in children <6 years old and in patients with intestinal obstruction.

5-HT₄ AGONISTS — Serotonin (5-HT) plays a major role in the regulation of GI motility, secretion, and sensation.[2] Agonism of 5-HT_4 receptors stimulates secretions and increases intestinal transit. **Tegaserod** *(Zelnorm)*, a partial 5-HT_4 receptor agonist was approved in 2002 for treatment of IBS-C, but it was withdrawn from the market in 2007 due to an increased risk of adverse cardiovascular events. Recently, however, an FDA advisory committee re-examined the data leading to the withdrawal and recommended a limited approval. Tegaserod is once again approved for treatment of IBS-C, but only in women <65 years old without a history of MI, angina, stroke, or transient ischemic attack.[34]

Adverse Effects – The most common adverse effects of tegaserod are headache, abdominal pain, nausea, diarrhea, flatulence, dyspepsia, and dizziness. Tegaserod is contraindicated for use in patients with a history of MI, stroke, transient ischemic attack, angina, ischemic colitis or other forms of intestinal ischemia, bowel obstruction, symptomatic gallbladder disease, suspected sphincter of Oddi dysfunction, or abdominal adhesions, and in those with moderate or severe hepatic impairment or severe or end-stage renal disease.

Drug Interactions – Tegaserod is a substrate of P-glycoprotein (P-gp); concurrent use with inhibitors of P-gp may increase systemic exposure to tegaserod.[21]

DRUGS FOR IBS-D

ANTIDIARRHEALS — The synthetic opioids loperamide *(Imodium A-D*, and generics; available OTC) and diphenoxylate/atropine *(Lomotil)* have been used to reduce stool frequency in patients with IBS-D, but they do not reduce global IBS symptoms such as discomfort and bloating.[1,2]

ANTIBIOTIC — **Rifaximin** *(Xifaxan)*, a minimally absorbed oral antibiotic FDA-approved for treatment of IBS-D,[35] is thought to alter gut microbiota and may reduce mucosal inflammation and visceral hypersensitivity. In two randomized, double-blind trials in a total of 1260 patients with IBS without constipation, significantly more patients who took rifaximin reported adequate relief of global IBS symptoms (41% vs 32% with placebo).[36] Repeat treatment, which is often required, has been shown to be safe and effective.[37]

Adverse Effects – In IBS-D clinical trials, the most common adverse effects of rifaximin were nausea (3%) and elevated ALT levels (2%). *Clostridioides (Clostridium) difficile*-associated colitis, creatine phosphokinase elevations, and myalgia have occurred rarely. Hypersensitivity reactions have been reported.

Drug Interactions – Rifaximin is a substrate of P-gp. Concomitant administration of cyclosporine, a P-gp inhibitor, resulted in an 83-fold increase in the Cmax and a 124-fold increase in the AUC of rifaximin. Other P-gp inhibitors may have a similar effect.[21] Whether such large increases in serum concentrations of the drug increase the incidence or severity of adverse effects is unknown. Changes in INR have been reported in patients concurrently taking warfarin and rifaximin.

BILE ACID SEQUESTRANTS — **Cholestyramine** (*Questran*, and others), **colestipol** (*Colestid*, and generics), and **colesevelam** (*Welchol*, and generics) have been used off-label to increase colonic transit time and improve IBS symptoms, but data are limited.[38]

Adverse Effects – Bile acid sequestrants can cause constipation, heartburn, nausea, eructation, flatulence and bloating, and can impair absorption of fat-soluble vitamins. Colesevelam is better tolerated than cholestyramine or colestipol.

Drug Interactions – Bile acid sequestrants can interfere with the absorption of fat-soluble vitamins and other oral drugs; they should be taken several hours apart.

OPIOID RECEPTOR AGONIST/ANTAGONIST — **Eluxadoline** (*Viberzi*), a mu-opioid receptor agonist and delta-opioid receptor antagonist, is FDA-approved for treatment of IBS-D.[39] Stimulation of mu-opioid receptors in the GI tract leads to decreased muscle contractility, inhibition of water and electrolyte secretion, and increased rectal sphincter tone. Antagonism of delta-opioid receptors in the gut may reduce iatrogenic constipation and abdominal pain. Systemic absorption of eluxadoline is minimal at therapeutic doses.

In two randomized, double-blind trials in a total of 2427 patients with IBS-D, the composite response rate at week 12 (a ≥30% improvement in abdominal pain score and an improvement in stool consistency from baseline on ≥50% of treatment days) was significantly higher with eluxadoline 75 mg (24% and 29%) and 100 mg (25% and 30%) than with placebo (17% and 16%).[40]

Adverse Effects – Eluxadoline can cause constipation, nausea, and abdominal pain. Sphincter of Oddi spasm and pancreatitis have been reported.[41] The drug is contraindicated in patients with a history of cholecystectomy, known or suspected biliary duct, pancreatic duct, or GI tract obstruction, sphincter of Oddi disease or dysfunction, severe hepatic impairment (Child-Pugh C), or a history of chronic or severe constipation, pancreatitis, or structural pancreatic disease. It is also contraindicated in patients who drink >3 alcoholic beverages per day; such patients are at increased risk for pancreatitis. Euphoria and feelings of drunkenness have been reported in clinical trials; eluxadoline is classified as a schedule IV controlled substance.

Drug Interactions – Coadministration of eluxadoline with other drugs that reduce GI motility, such as anticholinergic drugs or systemically active opioids, could result in additive effects and should be avoided. Loperamide can be used occasionally with eluxadoline for acute treatment of severe diarrhea, but it should be stopped if constipation occurs.

Eluxadoline is a substrate of organic anion transporting polypeptide (OATP) 1B1 and an inhibitor of OATP1B1 and breast cancer resistance protein (BCRP). Drugs that are substrates of both transporters, such as rosuvastatin (*Crestor*, and generics), should be administered at the lowest effective dose if taken with eluxadoline.

5-HT$_3$ ANTAGONISTS — Serotonin (5-HT) plays a major role in the regulation of GI motility, secretion, and sensation.[2] Antagonism of 5-HT$_3$ receptors has been shown to decrease pain and slow intestinal transit.

Alosetron (*Lotronex*, and generics), a 5-HT$_3$ receptor antagonist, relieves abdominal pain and discomfort, decreases bowel urgency and stool frequency, and improves stool consistency.[42] After initial approval of alosetron for IBS-D, it was withdrawn from the market in 2000 because of reports of severe constipation and ischemic colitis. It was reintroduced in 2002 with new labeling recommending a 50% lower starting dose and limiting its use to women with severe chronic IBS-D refractory to conventional therapies. In a randomized, double-blind trial comparing alosetron (0.5 mg daily, 1 mg daily, or 1 mg twice daily) to placebo in 705 women with severe IBS-D, global IBS symptoms improved significantly with all three doses of alosetron (50.8%, 48.0%, and 42.9%, respectively, vs 30.7% with placebo).[43]

Ondansetron (*Zofran*, and generics), a 5-HT$_3$ receptor antagonist, is FDA-approved for prevention of chemotherapy-induced and postoperative nausea and vomiting. In a randomized, double-blind, placebo-controlled, crossover study in 120 patients with IBS-D, ondansetron (median dose of 4 mg daily) decreased the frequency of loose stools and reduced urgency and bloating, but it did not significantly improve pain scores.[44]

Adverse Effects – Constipation is the most common adverse effect reported with both drugs in patients with IBS-D. Ischemic colitis is a rare but serious complication associated with alosetron.[45]

Drug Interactions – Alosetron is a substrate of CYP1A2 and 3A4. It is contraindicated for use with the strong CYP1A2 inhibitor fluvoxamine and use with moderate 1A2 inhibitors or 3A4 inhibitors should be avoided.[21] **Ondansetron** can prolong the QT interval and cause serotonin syndrome; patients taking other drugs that also prolong the QT interval or have serotonergic activity should be closely monitored.

1. AC Ford et al. American College of Gastroenterology monograph on management of irritable bowel syndrome. Am J Gastroenterol 2018; 113(Suppl 2):1.
2. AC Ford et al. Irritable bowel syndrome. N Engl J Med 2017; 376:2566.
3. SL Eswaran et al. A randomized controlled trial comparing the low FODMAPS diet vs. modified NICE guidelines in US adults with IBS-D. Am J Gastroenterol 2016; 111:1824.
4. SJ Shepherd et al. Short-chain carbohydrates and functional gastrointestinal disorders. Am J Gastroenterol 2013; 108:707.
5. JR Biesiekierski et al. Gluten causes gastrointestinal symptoms in subjects without celiac disease: a double-blind randomized placebo-controlled trial. Am J Gastroenterol 2011; 106:508.
6. JR Biesiekierski et al. No effects of gluten in patients with self-reported non-celiac gluten sensitivity after dietary reduction of fermentable, poorly absorbed, short-chain carbohydrates. Gastroenterology 2013; 145:320.
7. J Dionne et al. A systematic review and meta-analysis evaluating the efficacy of a gluten-free diet and a low FODMAPs diet in treating symptoms of irritable bowel syndrome. Am J Gastroenterol 2018; 113:1290.
8. C Zhou et al. Exercise therapy of patients with irritable bowel syndrome: a systematic review of randomized controlled trials. Neurogastroenterol Motil 2019; 31:e13461.
9. E Johannesson et al. Physical activity improves symptoms in irritable bowel syndrome: a randomized controlled trial. Am J Gastroenterol 2011; 106:915.
10. D Schumann et al. Effect of yoga in the therapy of irritable bowel syndrome: a systematic review. Clin Gastroenterol Hepatol 2016; 14:1720.
11. D Schumann et al. Randomised clinical trial: yoga vs a low-FODMAP diet in patients with irritable bowel syndrome. Aliment Pharmacol Ther 2018; 47:203.
12. N Nagarajan et al. The role of fiber supplementation in the treatment of irritable bowel syndrome: a systematic review and meta-analysis. Eur J Gastroenterol Hepatol 2015; 27:1002.
13. S Merat et al. The effect of enteric-coated, delayed-release peppermint oil on irritable bowel syndrome. Dig Dis Sci 2010; 55:1385.
14. ZZRM Weerts et al. Efficacy and safety of peppermint oil in a randomized, double-blind trial of patients with irritable bowel syndrome. Gastroenterology 2020; 158:123.
15. M Rajilić-Stojanović et al. Intestinal microbiota and diet in IBS: causes, consequences, or epiphenomena? Am J Gastroenterol 2015; 110:278.
16. AC Ford et al. Efficacy of prebiotics, probiotics, and synbiotics in irritable bowel syndrome and chronic idiopathic constipation: systematic review and meta-analysis. Am J Gastroenterol 2014; 109:1547.
17. Probiotics revisited. Med Lett Drugs Ther 2013; 55:3.
18. AC Ford et al. Effect of antidepressants and psychological therapies in irritable bowel syndrome: an updated systematic review and meta-analysis. Am J Gastroenterol 2019; 114:21.

19. HA Everitt et al. Assessing telephone-delivered cognitive-behavioural therapy (CBT) and web-delivered CBT versus treatment as usual in irritable bowel syndrome (ACTIB): a multicentre randomised trial. Gut 2019; 68:1613.

20. L Ruepert et al. Bulking agents, antispasmodics and antidepressants for the treatment of irritable bowel syndrome. Cochrane Database Syst Rev 2011; 8:CD003460.

21. Inhibitors and inducers of CYP enzymes and P-glycoprotein. Med Lett Drugs Ther 2019 November 6 (epub). Available at: medicalletter.org/downloads/CYP_PGP_Tables.pdf.

22. Drugs for depression. Med Lett Drugs Ther 2020; 62:25.

23. YA Saito et al. Randomised clinical trial: pregabalin vs placebo for irritable bowel syndrome. Aliment Pharmacol Ther 2019; 49:389.

24. RW Chapman et al. Randomized clinical trial: macrogol/PEG 3350 plus electrolytes for treatment of patients with constipation associated with irritable bowel syndrome. Am J Gastroenterol 2013; 108:1508.

25. Lubiprostone (Amitiza) for irritable bowel syndrome with constipation. Med Lett Drugs Ther 2008; 50:53.

26. DA Drossman et al. Clinical trial: lubiprostone in patients with constipation-associated irritable bowel syndrome - results of two randomized, placebo-controlled studies. Aliment Pharmacol Ther 2009; 29:329.

27. FDA. Medical Review: Lubiprostone. Available at: http://bit.ly/338eu7d. Accessed March 12, 2020.

28. Linaclotide (Linzess) for constipation. Med Lett Drugs Ther 2012; 54:91.

29. S Rao et al. A 12-week, randomized, controlled trial with a 4-week randomized withdrawal period to evaluate the efficacy and safety of linaclotide in irritable bowel syndrome with constipation. Am J Gastroenterol 2012; 107:1714.

30. WD Chey et al. Linaclotide for irritable bowel syndrome with constipation: a 26-week, randomized, double-blind, placebo-controlled trial to evaluate efficacy and safety. Am J Gastroenterol 2012; 107:1702.

31. DM Brenner et al. Efficacy, safety, and tolerability of plecanatide in patients with irritable bowel syndrome with constipation: results of two phase 3 randomized clinical trials. Am J Gastroenterol 2018; 113:735.

32. A Munjal et al. Update on pharmacotherapy for irritable bowel syndrome. Curr Gastroenterol Rep 2019; 21:25.

33. WD Chey et al. Efficacy of tenapanor in treating patients with irritable bowel syndrome with constipation: a 12-week, placebo-controlled phase 3 trial (T3MPO-1). Am J Gastroenterol 2020; 115:281.

34. In brief: tegaserod (Zelnorm) returns. Med Lett Drugs Ther 2019; 61:72.

35. Rifaximin (Xifaxan) for irritable bowel syndrome with diarrhea. Med Lett Drugs Ther 2015; 57:109.

36. M Pimentel et al. Rifaximin therapy for patients with irritable bowel syndrome without constipation. N Engl J Med 2011; 364:22.

37. A Lembo et al. Repeat treatment with rifaximin is safe and effective in patients with diarrhea-predominant irritable bowel syndrome. Gastroenterology 2016; 151:1113.

38. M Camilleri et al. Effect of colesevelam on faecal bile acids and bowel functions in diarrhoea-predominant irritable bowel syndrome. Aliment Pharmacol Ther 2015; 41:438.

39. Eluxadoline (Viberzi) for irritable bowel syndrome with diarrhea. Med Lett Drugs Ther 2016; 58:4.
40. AJ Lembo et al. Eluxadoline for irritable bowel syndrome with diarrhea. N Engl J Med 2016; 374:242.
41. In brief: pancreatitis with eluxadoline (Viberzi) in patients without a gallbladder. Med Lett Drugs Ther 2017; 59:70.
42. Alosetron (Lotronex) revisited. Med Lett Drugs Ther 2002; 44:67.
43. R Krause et al. A randomized, double-blind, placebo-controlled study to assess efficacy and safety of 0.5 mg and 1 mg alosetron in women with severe diarrhea-predominant IBS. Am J Gastroenterol 2007; 102:1709.
44. K Garsed et al. A randomised trial of ondansetron for the treatment of irritable bowel syndrome with diarrhoea. Gut 2014; 63:1617.
45. K Tong et al. A 9-year evaluation of temporal trends in alosetron postmarketing safety under the risk management program. Therap Adv Gastroenterol 2013; 6:344.

DRUGS FOR
Menopausal Symptoms

Original publication date – August 2020 (revised October 2020)

The primary symptoms of menopause are genitourinary (genitourinary syndrome of menopause; GSM) and vasomotor (VMS). Vulvovaginal atrophy can cause vaginal burning, irritation and dryness, dyspareunia, and dysuria, and increase the risk of urinary tract infections. Vasomotor symptoms ("hot flashes") cause daytime discomfort and night sweats that may disrupt sleep. Hormone therapy is the most effective treatment for both genitourinary and vasomotor symptoms.[1,2]

Hormone therapy is contraindicated in women with unexplained vaginal bleeding, severe active liver disease, prior estrogen-sensitive malignancies (breast, endometrial, and possibly ovarian cancer), coronary heart disease, hypertriglyceridemia, stroke, or a personal or family history of thromboembolic disease.[2]

GENITOURINARY SYNDROME
OF MENOPAUSE

NONHORMONAL THERAPY — Over-the-counter (OTC) non-hormonal vaginal moisturizers and lubricants are generally tried first for treatment of genitourinary symptoms. Vaginal hormone therapy is recommended for women who have insufficient symptom relief with nonhormonal OTC products.

Summary: Drugs for Menopausal Symptoms

► Estrogen is the most effective treatment for both genitourinary and vasomotor symptoms.
► Low-dose vaginal estrogen products are preferred for treatment of the genito-urinary syndrome of menopause (GSM). Addition of a progestogen is generally not necessary.
► The oral estrogen agonist/antagonist ospemifene and the intravaginal steroid prasterone are alternatives to estrogen for women with GSM who are unwilling or unable to use an estrogen.
► Systemic estrogen formulations are preferred for treatment of vasomotor symptoms (VMS). Women with an intact uterus who use a systemic estrogen should also receive a progestogen or bazedoxifene (available in combination with conjugated estrogens) for endometrial protection.
► Nonhormonal therapies such as an antidepressant are alternatives to hormonal therapy in women with VMS.

ESTROGEN — Low-dose vaginal estrogen products are recommended for women with genitourinary syndrome of menopause without vaso-motor symptoms (see Table 1). All low-dose vaginal estrogen products are similarly effective for treatment of vulvovaginal atrophy. Systemic effects are minimal, and addition of a progestogen to protect against endometrial hyperplasia and cancer is generally not required.[2,3]

OSPEMIFENE — The selective estrogen receptor modulator (SERM) ospemifene *(Osphena)*, an oral estrogen agonist/antagonist that has agonist effects on vaginal epithelium and the endometrium and anti-estrogenic effects in animal models of breast cancer, is FDA-approved for treatment of moderate to severe vaginal dryness and moderate to severe dyspareunia due to vulvovaginal atrophy. It can be used as an oral alternative to a vaginal estrogen. How ospemifene compares in efficacy to vaginal estrogens is unclear.

Ospemifene reduces the severity of dyspareunia and improves other symptoms associated with genitourinary syndrome of menopause, but hot flashes, vaginal discharge, muscle spasms, hyperhidrosis, and venous thromboembolism can occur.[4] Endometrial thickening and uterine polyps can also occur; no cases of endometrial hyperplasia or carcinoma have been reported with use of ospemifene for up to 52 weeks.[5,6] Its safety in women with or at risk for breast cancer remains to be established.

Postmenopausal women with an intact uterus who can be followed closely for vaginal bleeding or spotting and do not have risk factors for endometrial cancer (obesity, hypertension, diabetes, nulliparity) could take ospemifene without a progestogen. For all others, addition of a progestogen should be considered.[7]

PRASTERONE — The steroid prasterone, also known as dehydro-epiandrosterone (DHEA), is FDA-approved as an intravaginal insert *(Intrarosa)* for treatment of moderate to severe dyspareunia due to vulvo-vaginal atrophy. DHEA is produced in the adrenal glands, gonads, and brain and converted intracellularly into active metabolites of estrogens and androgens. DHEA is also available by prescription as a compounded vaginal cream for vulvovaginal atrophy and over the counter as an oral dietary supplement.[8] Prasterone can be used as an alternative to a vaginal estrogen. Vaginal discharge and abnormal Pap smears have been the most common adverse effects. Studies in women with or at risk for breast cancer are limited.[9] How prasterone compares in efficacy to vaginal estrogens remains to be determined.

VASOMOTOR MENOPAUSAL SYMPTOMS

ESTROGEN — Systemic estrogen (oral, transdermal, and vaginal; see Table 2) is the most effective treatment for vasomotor symptoms, reducing hot flashes by 50-100% within 4 weeks,[10] but its use may increase the risk of endometrial hyperplasia and cancer, breast cancer (at least when taken with medroxyprogesterone[11]), venous thromboembo-lism, coronary artery disease, and stroke, especially in women ≥60 years old or >10 years past the onset of menopause. Transdermal estrogens are as effective as oral estrogens, and they are generally considered less likely to cause thromboembolic and other systemic adverse effects.[12,13]

Table 1. Drugs for Genitourinary Syndrome of Menopause (GSM)[1]	
Drug	**Some Formulations**
Vaginal	
Estradiol – *Estring* (Pfizer)	2 mg ring (7.5 mcg/day)
Estradiol – *Imvexxy* (Therapeutics MD)	4, 10 mcg inserts
Vagifem (Novo Nordisk)	10 mcg insert[4]
generic	
Yuvafem (Amneal)[5]	10 mcg insert[4]
Estradiol – *Estrace* (Abbvie)	0.1 mg/gram cream
generic	
Conjugated estrogens – *Premarin* (Pfizer)	0.625 mg/gram cream
Prasterone – *Intrarosa* (Millicent)	6.5 mg insert
Oral	
Ospemifene – *Osphena* (Duchesnay)	60 mg tabs

1. Low-dose vaginal estrogen products are preferred for women with only genitourinary symptoms. Recommended doses of *Estring, Imvexxy,* and *Vagifem* and the 0.5-gram dose of *Premarin* are considered low doses. Addition of a progestogen is generally not necessary for low-dose vaginal estrogen products (CA Stuenkel et al. J Clin Endocrinol Metab 2015; 100:3975; JE Manson et al. Menopause 2014; 21:911).
2. Approximate WAC for 90 days' maintenance treatment with the lowest strength. WAC = wholesaler acquisition cost or manufacturer's published price to wholesalers; WAC represents a published catalogue or list price and may not represent an actual transactional price. Source: AnalySource® Monthly. July 5, 2020. Reprinted with permission by First Databank, Inc. All rights reserved. ©2020. www.fdbhealth.com/policies/drug-pricing-policy.

PROGESTOGENS — Endometrial hyperplasia has been reported in >20% of women taking an unopposed systemic estrogen for >1 year; the risk is closely related to the dosage and duration of treatment. To reduce the risk of endometrial hyperplasia and cancer, women with an intact uterus treated with a systemic estrogen should also receive a progestogen or possibly the SERM bazedoxifene, which is only available in a fixed-dose combination with conjugated estrogens. Adding a progestogen to a systemic estrogen increases the risk of breast cancer, thromboembolism, and cardiovascular disease. Micronized progesterone or (off-label) a levonorgestrel-releasing IUD may be less likely than medroxyprogesterone to increase these risks.[13]

CONJUGATED ESTROGENS/SERM — A fixed-dose combination of conjugated estrogens and the SERM bazedoxifene *(Duavee)* is FDA-approved for treatment of moderate to severe vasomotor symptoms in

Usual Dosage	Cost[2]
7.5 mcg/day[3]	$475.60
4 or 10 mcg once/day x 2 wks, then 2x/wk	572.40
10 mcg once/day x 2 wks, then 2x/wk	521.30
	465.60
	160.30
2-4 g once/day x 1-2 wks, then 1-2 g once/day x 1-2 wks[6]	344.80[7]
	271.00[7]
0.5-2 g once/day x 3 wks followed by 7 days off, or 0.5 g 2x/wk	392.20[8]
6.5 mg once/day at bedtime	682.40
60 mg once/day	680.40

3. The ring should remain in place continuously for 90 days. A new ring can be inserted after 90 days, but the need for continued treatment should be reassessed at 3- or 6-month intervals.
4. Supplied as single-use, disposable applicators containing one estradiol tablet.
5. Branded generic of *Vagifem*.
6. 1 gram one to three times each week can be used after vaginal mucosa has been restored.
7. Cost of one 42.5-gram tube.
8. Cost of one 30-gram tube.

postmenopausal women with an intact uterus and for prevention of osteoporosis in postmenopausal women.[14] Bazedoxifene has estrogen-like effects on vasomotor symptoms and antiestrogen effects on the uterus. In clinical trials, the combination reduced the severity and frequency of hot flashes compared to placebo. The risks of venous thromboembolism, coronary heart disease, breast cancer, and ischemic stroke with long-term use of *Duavee* remain to be determined.[15]

BIOIDENTICAL HORMONES — "Bioidentical" hormones are exogenous hormone products that are chemically identical to endogenous hormones such as estradiol and progesterone. The practice of compounding personalized doses of bioidentical hormones such as estriol has increased in recent years. These preparations are not regulated by the FDA and their potency and purity can vary. There is no acceptable

Table 2. Drugs for Vasomotor Symptoms (VMS)

Drug	Some Formulations
Oral Estrogens[2]	
Conjugated estrogens[3] – *Premarin* (Pfizer)[4]	0.3, 0.45, 0.625, 0.9, 1.25 mg tabs
Estradiol[4] – generic *Estrace* (Abbvie)	0.5, 1, 2 mg tabs
Esterified estrogen – *Menest* (Monarch)[4]	0.3, 0.625, 1.25, 2.5 mg tabs
Oral Progestogens	
Progesterone (micronized) – generic *Prometrium* (Virtus)	100, 200 mg caps
Medroxyprogesterone – generic *Provera* (Pfizer)	2.5, 5, 10 mg tabs
Oral Estrogen/Progestogen Combinations	
Conjugated estrogens[3]/ medroxyprogesterone – *Prempro* (Pfizer)[4,6]	0.3/1.5, 0.45/1.5, 0.625/2.5, 0.625/5 mg tabs
Estradiol/drospirenone – *Angeliq* (Bayer)[7]	0.5/0.25, 1/0.5 mg tabs
Estradiol/norethindrone[8] – *Activella* (Amneal)[7]	0.5/0.1, 1/0.5 mg tabs
Estradiol/progesterone – *Bijuva* (Therapeutics MD)	1/100 mg caps
Ethinyl estradiol/norethindrone[8] – *Femhrt* (Abbvie)	2.5 mcg/0.5 mg tabs
Oral Estrogen/Selective Estrogen Reuptake Modulator (SERM)	
Conjugated estrogens[3]/bazedoxifene – *Duavee* (Pfizer)	0.45/20 mg tabs
Transdermal Estrogens[2]	
Estradiol patches[4,8] – *Alora* (Abbvie)	0.025, 0.05, 0.075, 0.1 mg/day patches
Climara (Bayer)	0.025, 0.0375, 0.05, 0.06, 0.075, 0.1 mg/day patches
Vivelle-DOT (Novartis)	0.025, 0.0375, 0.05, 0.075, 0.1 mg/day patches

1. Approximate WAC for 30 days' or 4 weeks' treatment at the lowest usual dosage. WAC = wholesaler acquisition cost or manufacturer's published price to wholesalers; WAC represents a published catalogue or list price and may not represent an actual transactional price. Source: AnalySource® Monthly. July 5, 2020. Reprinted with permission from First Databank, Inc. All rights reserved. ©2020. www.fdbhealth.com/policies/drug-pricing-policy.
2. For women with an intact uterus, addition of a progestogen is recommended.
3. Conjugated estrogens are derived from the urine of pregnant mares.

Drugs for Menopausal Symptoms

Usual Dosage	Cost[1]
0.3-0.625 mg PO once/day	$177.00
0.5-1 mg PO once/day	0.90
	163.50
0.625-1.25 mg PO once/day	74.90
100 mg PO once/day[5]	25.90
	316.70
5-10 mg PO once/day x 12-14 days/month	2.60
	45.20
0.3/1.5-0.625/5 mg PO once/day	202.80
0.5/0.25 or 1/0.5 mg PO once/day	186.20
0.5/0.1 or 1/0.5 mg PO once/day	255.60
1/100 mg PO once/day	214.50
2.5 mcg/0.5 mg or 5 mcg/1 mg PO once/day	156.90
0.45/20 mg PO once/day	185.60
0.05 mg/day patch 2x/wk	113.00
0.05 mg/day patch once/wk	138.40
0.05 mg/day patch 2x/wk	121.30

4. Also FDA-approved for treatment of vulvar and vaginal atrophy associated with menopause.
5. 200 mg PO once/day x 12 days per 28-day cycle is an alternative.
6. Also available as *Premphase*, which contains 14 combination tablets and 14 conjugated estrogen tablets.
7. The 1/0.5 mg tabs are also FDA-approved for treatment of vulvar and vaginal atrophy associated with menopause.
8. Available generically.

Continued on next page

Table 2. Drugs for Vasomotor Symptoms (VMS) (continued)	
Drug	**Some Formulations**
Transdermal Estrogens[2] (continued)	
Estradiol gel – *EstroGel* (Ascend Therapeutics)[4]	0.75 mg/actuation (30 doses/unit)[9]
Divigel (Osmotica)	0.25, 0.5, 0.75, 1, 1.25 mg/packets
Elestrin (Meda)	0.52 mg/actuation (100 doses/unit)[11]
Estradiol transdermal spray – *Evamist* (Perrigo)	1.53 mg/spray (56 sprays/unit)
Vaginal Estrogen[2]	
Estradiol intravaginal ring – *Femring* (Millicent)[4]	0.05, 0.1 mg/day vaginal rings
Transdermal Estrogen/Progestin Combinations	
Estradiol/levonorgestrel – *Climara Pro* (Bayer)	0.045/0.015 mg/day patches
Estradiol/norethindrone – *CombiPatch* (Noven Therapeutics)[4]	0.05/0.14, 0.05/0.25 mg/day patches
Selective Serotonin Reuptake Inhibitor (SSRI)	
Paroxetine mesylate – generic *Brisdelle* (Sebela)	7.5 mg caps

9. Each actuation delivers 1.25 g of gel containing 0.75 mg of estradiol.
10. Cost of one 50-g bottle.
11. Each metered dose delivers 0.87 g of gel, which contains 0.52 mg of estradiol.
12. Cost of one 28-g bottle.
13. Cost of one 8.1-mL bottle.

evidence that bioidentical hormones are more effective or safer than conjugated or fully synthetic hormones.[16,17]

NONHORMONAL DRUGS — Antidepressants – In randomized, placebo-controlled trials, off-label use of antidepressants has produced modest improvements in vasomotor symptoms compared to placebo.[18,19]

A low-dose formulation of the selective serotonin reuptake inhibitor (SSRI) **paroxetine mesylate** *(Brisdelle)* is the only nonhormonal therapy that is FDA-approved for treatment of moderate to severe vasomotor

Usual Dosage	Cost[1]
0.75 mg applied once/day	$127.40[10]
0.25-1 mg applied once/day	87.00
0.52 mg applied once/day	107.50[12]
2 sprays once/day	123.80[13]
0.05 mg/day[14]	531.50[15]
0.045/0.015 mg/day patch once/wk	221.90
0.05/0.14 or 0.05/0.25 mg/day patch 2x/wk[16]	207.40
7.5 mg PO once/day at hs	151.20
	211.90

14. The ring should remain in place continuously for 90 days. A new ring can be inserted after 90 days, but the need for continued treatment should be reassessed at 3- or 6-month intervals.
15. Cost of one ring.
16. Can also be used in combination with an estradiol-only transdermal system that is worn for the first 14 days of a 28-day cycle and is then replaced by *CombiPatch* every 3-4 days for the remaining 14 days.

symptoms. It has reduced the severity and frequency (by 6-10/day) of hot flashes compared to placebo, but it can cause headache, lethargy, nausea, and vomiting. *Brisdelle* has not been reported to cause weight gain or sexual dysfunction, both of which occur with higher doses of paroxetine.[20] No trials are available directly comparing *Brisdelle* with other paroxetine formulations or with other antidepressants for treatment of vasomotor symptoms.[21] Many SSRIs and serotonin-norepinephrine reuptake inhibitors (SNRIs) can interfere with the CYP2D6-mediated conversion of tamoxifen to its most active metabolite; *Brisdelle* should not be used in women who are taking tamoxifen.

In one study, the SSRI **escitalopram** (*Lexapro*, and generics), the SNRI **venlafaxine** (*Effexor XR*, and generics), and low-dose oral estradiol were about equally effective in reducing the frequency of hot flashes (by about 50% vs 30% with placebo).[22]

Other Drugs – The anticonvulsant **gabapentin** (*Neurontin*, and others) has also been reported to reduce hot flashes (off-label use). Evidence supporting the use of **pregabalin** (*Lyrica*, and others) for reducing vasomotor symptoms is lacking.[23]

In one study, the benzodiazepine receptor agonist **eszopiclone** (*Lunesta*, and generics) improved sleep, depression, anxiety symptoms, and night-time (but not daytime) vasomotor symptoms in perimenopausal and early postmenopausal women (off-label use).[24]

The anticholinergic drug **oxybutynin** (*Ditropan XL*, and generics) has been shown to reduce the frequency and severity of hot flashes in healthy menopausal women and in those with a history of breast cancer (off-label use).[25] Long-term use of anticholinergic drugs may increase the risk of dementia and is not recommended.[26]

The alpha$_2$-adrenergic agonist clonidine has been shown to be effective for treatment of vasomotor symptoms, but it is no longer preferred because of its adverse effects, modest efficacy, and the availability of other more effective nonhormonal drugs.

ALTERNATIVE THERAPIES — Complementary and alternative therapies are widely used for management of vasomotor symptoms in postmenopausal women, but well-established safety and efficacy data are lacking.[27]

Phytoestrogens (isoflavones, coumestans, or lignans) are plant-derived nonsteroidal compounds that bind to estrogen receptors and have both estrogenic and antiestrogenic properties. A meta-analysis found that ingesting soy-containing foods and soy extracts (both sources of isoflavones) was associated with a modest reduction in hot flashes and vaginal dryness.[28] A meta-analysis of 9 randomized, controlled trials suggested that flaxseed can relieve vasomotor symptoms, but the results of individual studies have been mixed.[29,30] In one randomized controlled trial, a purified pollen extract taken orally was significantly more effective than placebo in relieving hot flashes.[31]

Black cohosh, an herbal supplement, has been claimed to improve vasomotor symptoms, but it was not more effective than placebo in a 1-year study in 351 symptomatic postmenopausal women.[32] Hepatic toxicity has been reported.[33]

Evening primrose oil, ginseng, dong quai, wild yam, red clover, and **acupuncture** have all been tried for treatment of vasomotor symptoms, but there is no acceptable evidence that any of them are effective for this indication.[34]

1. A Stuenkel et al. Treatment of symptoms of the menopause: an Endocrine Society clinical practice guideline. J Clin Endocrinol Metab 2015; 100:3975.
2. The NAMS 2017 Hormone Therapy Position Statement Advisory Panel. The 2017 hormone therapy position statement of The North American Menopause Society. Menopause 2017; 24:728.
3. CJ Crandall et al. Breast cancer, endometrial cancer, and cardiovascular events in participants who used vaginal estrogen in the Women's Health Initiative Observational Study. Menopause 2018; 25:11.
4. Ospemifene (Osphena) for dyspareunia. Med Lett Drugs Ther 2013; 55:55.
5. JA Simon et al. One-year long-term safety extension study of ospemifene for the treatment of vulvar and vaginal atrophy in postmenopausal women with a uterus. Menopause 2013; 20:418.
6. GD Constantine et al. Endometrial safety of ospemifene: results of the phase 2/3 clinical development program. Menopause 2015; 22:36.
7. Addendum: Ospemifene (Osphena) for dyspareunia. Med Lett Drugs Ther 2013; 55:84.
8. Prasterone (Intrarosa) for dyspareunia. Med Lett Drugs Ther 2017; 59:149.
9. DL Barton et al. Systemic and local effects of vaginal dehydroepiandrosterone (DHEA): NCCTG N10C1 (Alliance). Support Cancer Care 2018; 26:1335.
10. AH MacLennan et al. Oral oestrogen and combined oestrogen/progestogen therapy versus placebo for hot flushes. Cochrane Database Syst Rev 2004; 4:CD002978.
11. RT Chlebowski et al. Association of menopausal hormone therapy with breast cancer incidence and mortality during long-term follow-up of the Women's Health Initiative randomized clinical trials. JAMA 2020; 324:369.

12 JL Shifren et al. Menopausal hormone therapy. JAMA 2019; 321:2458.

13. RH Cobin et al. American Association of Clinical Endocrinologists and American College of Endocrinology position statement on menopause-2017 update. Endocr Pract 2017; 23:869.

14. Drugs for postmenopausal osteoporosis. Med Lett Drugs Ther 2020; 62:105.

15. Conjugated estrogens/bazedoxifene (Duavee) for menopausal symptoms and prevention of osteoporosis. Med Lett Drugs Ther 2014; 56:33.

16. N Santoro et al. Compounded bioidentical hormones in endocrinology practice: an Endocrine Society scientific statement. J Clin Endocrinol Metab 2016; 101:1318.

17. AM Gaudard et al. Bioidentical hormones for women with vasomotor symptoms. Cochrane Database Syst Rev 2016; 8:CD010407.

18. DL Barton et al. Phase III, placebo-controlled trial of three doses of citalopram for the treatment of hot flashes: NCCTG trial N05C9. J Clin Oncol 2010; 28:3278.

19. EW Freeman et al. Efficacy of escitalopram for hot flashes in healthy menopausal women: a randomized controlled trial. JAMA 2011; 305:267.

20. DJ Portman et al. Effects of low-dose paroxetine 7.5 mg on weight and sexual function during treatment of vasomotor symptoms associated with menopause. Menopause 2014; 21:1082.

21. Paroxetine (Brisdelle) for hot flashes. Med Lett Drugs Ther 2013; 55:85.

22. SD Reed et al. Lights on MsFLASH: a review of contributions. Menopause 2020; 27:473.

23. D Shan et al. Efficacy and safety of gabapentin and pregabalin in patients with vasomotor symptoms: a systematic review and meta-analysis. Am J Obstet Gynecol 2019; 222:564.

24. H Joffe et al. Eszopiclone improves insomnia and depressive and anxious symptoms in perimenopausal and postmenopausal women with hot flashes: a randomized, double-blinded, placebo-controlled crossover trial. Am J Obstet Gynecol 2010; 202:171.

25. RA Leon-Ferre et al. Oxybutynin vs placebo for hot flashes in women with or without breast cancer: a randomized, double-blind clinical trial (ACCRU SC-1603). JNCI Cancer Spectrum 2020; 4:pkz088.

26. Oxybutynin for hot flashes in women with breast cancer. Med Lett Drugs Ther 2019; 61:30.

27. PP Guo et al. Complementary and alternative medicine for natural and treatment-induced vasomotor symptoms: an overview of systematic reviews and meta-analyses. Complement Ther Clin Pract 2019; 36:181.

28. OH Franco et al. Use of plant-based therapies and menopausal symptoms: a systematic review and meta-analysis. JAMA 2016; 315:2554.

29. S Dodin et al. The effects of flaxseed dietary supplement on lipid profile, bone mineral density, and symptoms in menopausal women: a randomized, double-blind, wheat germ placebo-controlled clinical trial. J Clin Endocrinol Metab 2005; 90:1390.

30. M Ghazanfarpour et al. Effects of flaxseed and *Hypericum perforatum* on hot flash, vaginal atrophy and estrogen-dependent cancers in menopausal women: a systematic review and meta-analysis. Avicenna J Phytomed 2016; 6:273.

31. K Winther et al. Femal, a herbal remedy made from pollen extracts, reduces hot flushes and improves quality of life in menopausal women: a randomized, placebo-controlled, parallel study. Climacteric 2005; 8:162.

32. SD Reed et al. Vaginal, endometrial, and reproductive hormone findings: randomized, placebo-controlled trial of black cohosh, multibotanical herbs, and dietary soy for

vasomotor symptoms: the Herbal Alternatives for Menopause (HALT) Study. Menopause 2008; 15:51.

33. AC Brown et al. Liver toxicity related to herbs and dietary supplements: online table of case reports. Part 2 of 5 series. Food Chem Toxicol 2017; 107:472.

34. NAMS. Nonhormonal management of menopause-associated vasomotor symptoms: 2015 position statement of The North American Menopause Society. Menopause 2015; 22:1155.

DRUGS FOR
Migraine

Original publication date – October 2020

ACUTE TREATMENT OF MIGRAINE

An oral nonopioid analgesic is often sufficient for acute treatment of mild to moderate migraine headache without severe nausea or vomiting. A triptan is the drug of choice for treatment of moderate to severe migraine headache pain in most patients without vascular disease.[1,2] Early treatment of pain when it is still mild to moderate in intensity improves headache response and reduces the risk of recurrence.

ANALGESICS — **Aspirin** and **acetaminophen,** used alone, together, and in combination with caffeine, and **nonsteroidal anti-inflammatory drugs (NSAIDs)** such as naproxen and ibuprofen are effective in relieving mild to moderate migraine headache.[3-5] Diclofenac is available in a powder for oral solution *(Cambia)* for treatment of migraine; it has a rapid onset of action (about 15 minutes).[6] An oral solution of celecoxib *(Elyxyb)* has been approved by the FDA, but has not yet been marketed.

Products that contain **butalbital**, caffeine, and aspirin (*Fiorinal*, and others) or acetaminophen (*Fioricet*, and others) are marketed for treatment of migraine despite limited evidence that butalbital is effective in relieving migraine pain. Oral combinations of aspirin or acetaminophen and an **opioid** can be effective for relief of migraine pain, but they can cause opioid adverse effects (e.g., nausea, drowsiness, constipation).

Regular use of butalbital or opioids can lead to medication overuse headache, tolerance, dependence, and addiction.

Pregnancy – Occasional use of acetaminophen during pregnancy is generally considered safe. Use of NSAIDs during the third trimester may cause premature closure of the ductus arteriosus and persistent pulmonary hypertension in the neonate, but these effects appear to be uncommon if the drug is stopped 6-8 weeks before delivery. Butalbital has been associated with congenital heart defects and should not be used during pregnancy.

TRIPTANS — The shorter-acting oral 5-$HT_{1B/1D}$ receptor agonists (triptans) **sumatriptan**, **almotriptan**, **eletriptan**, **rizatriptan**, and **zolmitriptan** are similar in efficacy.[7] Onset of pain relief generally occurs 30-60 minutes after administration. The longer-acting oral triptans **naratriptan** and **frovatriptan** are generally better tolerated than shorter-acting triptans, but they have a slower onset of action and lower initial response rates. Patients who do not respond to one triptan may respond to another.

Patients with nausea or vomiting may not be able to take an oral triptan. Intranasal triptan formulations are faster-acting than oral tablets. Sumatriptan plasma concentrations peak faster and at higher levels with use of the nasal powder *(Onzetra Xsail)* than with use of nasal spray formulations.[8] Subcutaneously administered sumatriptan relieves pain faster and more effectively than other triptan formulations, but it causes more adverse effects.[9]

An oral fixed-dose combination of sumatriptan and naproxen (*Treximet*, and generics) is more effective in relieving moderate or severe migraine headache than either of its components alone.[10]

Recurrence – About 20-40% of moderate to severe migraine headaches recur within 24 hours after treatment with a triptan. Early treatment of an attack reduces recurrence rates. Recurrences may respond to a second dose of the triptan.

Summary: Drugs for Migraine

Acute Treatment

- An oral nonopioid analgesic is often sufficient for mild to moderate migraine headache.
- A triptan is the drug of choice for moderate to severe migraine headache pain in most patients without vascular disease.
- The shorter-acting oral triptans sumatriptan, almotriptan, eletriptan, rizatriptan, and zolmitriptan are similar in efficacy, speed of onset, and duration of action.
- Intranasal triptan formulations have a faster onset of action than oral triptans. Subcutaneous sumatriptan is the fastest-acting and most effective triptan formulation, but it causes the most adverse effects.
- The CGRP receptor antagonists rimegepant and ubrogepant appear to be less effective than triptans, but they can be used in patients with vascular disease.
- The 5-HT$_{1F}$ receptor agonist lasmiditan can also be used in patients with vascular disease. It has not been compared directly with triptans or CGRP receptor antagonists.
- Use of opioid- or butalbital-containing products for migraine treatment is not recommended.

Preventive Treatment

- Beta blockers and the antiseizure drugs topiramate and valproate are effective for prevention of migraine, but may be difficult to tolerate.
- A CGRP antibody can be tried if oral drugs are ineffective or poorly tolerated.

Adverse Effects – Tingling, flushing, dizziness, drowsiness, fatigue, and a feeling of heaviness, tightness, or pressure in the chest can occur with all triptans, but most commonly with subcutaneous sumatriptan. A burning sensation at the injection site is also common with subcutaneous sumatriptan. Intranasal triptan formulations can leave an unpleasant after-taste. CNS symptoms such as somnolence and weakness are commonly reported following triptan therapy, but they may be part of the migraine attack, unmasked by the successful treatment of pain, rather than adverse effects of the drug. Sumatriptan and naratriptan are contraindicated for use in patients with severe hepatic impairment. Naratriptan is also contra-indicated in patients with severe renal impairment.

Angina, myocardial infarction, cardiac arrhythmia, stroke, seizure, and death have occurred rarely with use of triptans.[11] All triptans are contra-indicated for use in patients with ischemic or vasospastic coronary artery disease, Wolff-Parkinson-White syndrome, peripheral vascular disease, ischemic bowel disease, uncontrolled hypertension, or a history of stroke or transient ischemic attack. They should be used with caution in patients with other significant risk factors for vascular disease, particularly diabetes.

Drug Interactions – Triptans should not be used within 24 hours of another triptan or an ergot because vasoconstriction could be additive. Concurrent use of monoamine oxidase (MAO) inhibitors and triptans can result in additive serotonergic effects. Use of sumatriptan, rizatriptan, or zolmitriptan within 2 weeks after an MAO-A inhibitor can result in increased serum concentrations of these triptans and is contraindicated. Propranolol increases serum concentrations of rizatriptan. Cimetidine increases serum concentrations of zolmitriptan. Inhibitors of CYP3A4 can increase serum concentrations of almotriptan and eletriptan; eletriptan should not be used within 72 hours after a strong CYP3A4 inhibitor.[12] Serotonin syndrome has been reported with concurrent use of triptans and serotonin reuptake inhibitors, but data from large observa-tional studies suggest that the risk is low.[13,14]

Pregnancy and Lactation – A population study in Norway found no association between triptan use during pregnancy and birth defects.[15] Levels of sumatriptan and eletriptan in breast milk are low and would not be expected to cause adverse effects in most breastfed infants.[16]

CGRP RECEPTOR ANTAGONISTS — Calcitonin gene-related peptide (CGRP) is a potent endogenous vasodilator and pain signal-enhancing neuromodulator. Serum levels of CGRP appear to increase during migraine attacks and IV administration of CGRP has induced migraine-like headaches in patients with a history of migraine.[17] Two small-molecule CGRP receptor antagonists, **rimegepant** *(Nurtec ODT)* and **ubrogepant** *(Ubrelvy)*, are FDA-approved for acute treatment of migraine in adults.[18,19] Both drugs appear to begin reducing migraine pain

Table 1. Triptan Pharmacology		
Drug	**Onset of Action**	**Half-Life**
Almotriptan	30-60 min	3-4 hrs
Eletriptan	30-60 min	~4 hrs
Frovatriptan	~2 hrs	~26 hrs
Naratriptan	1-3 hrs	~6 hrs
Rizatriptan	30-60 min	2-3 hrs

Sumatriptan – tablets
   nasal spray and powder
   subcutaneous injection
	30-60 min
	10-15 min
	~10 min
		~2 hrs

Zolmitriptan – tablets nasal spray	30-60 min 10-15 min	2-3 hrs

within 60 minutes. In clinical trials, about 20% of patients who received either drug were free of headache pain 2 hours post-dose, compared to about 10% who received placebo. Rimegepant has a longer half-life than ubrogepant (~11 hours vs 5-7 hours). No trials directly comparing the two drugs with each other or with triptans are available. CGRP receptor antagonists appear to be less effective than triptans, but they can be used in patients with vascular disease.

Adverse Effects – Both ubrogepant and rimegepant were well tolerated in clinical trials. Nausea and somnolence occurred in <5% of patients. CGRP receptor antagonists do not have vasoconstrictive effects and have not been associated with medication overuse headache.

Drug Interactions – Both ubrogepant and rimegepant are metabolized primarily by CYP3A4 and are substrates of P-glycoprotein (P-gp) and breast cancer resistance protein (BCRP). Concurrent use of these drugs with strong inhibitors or inducers of CYP3A4 or with inhibitors of P-gp or BCRP should be avoided.[12]

Pregnancy and Lactation – Rimegepant and ubrogepant have not been studied in pregnant or lactating women.

Table 2. Some Drugs for Acute Treatment of Migraine

Drug	Some Formulations
Triptans	
Almotriptan[3] – generic	6.25, 12.5 mg tabs
Eletriptan – generic *Relpax* (Pfizer)	20, 40 mg tabs
Frovatriptan – generic *Frova* (Endo)	2.5 mg tabs
Naratriptan – generic *Amerge* (GSK)	1, 2.5 mg tabs

Rizatriptan[5] – generic
 	
  Maxalt (Merck)
  Maxalt-MLT
	5, 10 mg tabs
	5, 10 mg orally disintegrating tabs
	10 mg tabs
	10 mg orally disintegrating tabs

Sumatriptan – generic
  Imitrex (GSK)
 	
  Onzetra Xsail (Avanir)
  Tosymra (Upsher-Smith)
  Zembrace SymTouch (Promius)
	25, 50, 100 mg tabs
	
	6 mg/0.5 mL vials
	4, 6 mg/0.5 mL auto-injector[9]
	5, 20 mg/0.1 mL nasal spray
	
	11 mg nasal powder capsules
	10 mg single-use nasal spray
	3 mg/0.5 mL auto-injector

Zolmitriptan – generic
 	
  Zomig (Amneal)
  Zomig-ZMT
  Zomig nasal spray[3]
	2.5, 5 mg tabs
	2.5, 5 mg orally disintegrating tabs
	2.5, 5 mg tabs
	2.5, 5 mg orally disintegrating tabs
	2.5, 5 mg/0.1 mL nasal spray

1. Dosage adjustments may be needed for renal or hepatic impairment or for drug interactions.
2. Approximate WAC for one dose at the lowest usual dosage. WAC = wholesaler acquisition cost or manufacturer's published price to wholesalers; WAC represents a published catalogue or list price and may not represent an actual transactional price. Source: AnalySource® Monthly. September 5, 2020. Reprinted with permission by First Databank, Inc. All rights reserved. ©2020. www.fdbhealth.com/policies/drug-pricing-policy.
3. Also approved for use in patients 12-17 years old.
4. Should be taken with fluids.
5. Also approved for use in patients 6-17 years old.

Usual Adult Dosage[1]	Cost[2]
6.25 or 12.5 mg PO; can be repeated after 2 hrs (max 25 mg/day)	$33.40
20 or 40 mg PO; can be repeated after 2 hrs (max 80 mg/day)	12.80
	65.30
2.5 mg PO; can be repeated after 2 hrs (max 7.5 mg/day)[4]	45.40
	97.70
2.5 mg PO; can be repeated after 4 hrs (max 5 mg/day)	9.60
	56.60
5 or 10 mg PO; can be repeated after 2 hrs (max 30 mg/day)[6,7]	2.60
	2.10
	36.60
	36.60
50 or 100 mg PO; can be repeated after 2 hrs (max 200 mg/day)	1.40/67.30[8]
6 mg SC; can be repeated after 1 hr (max 12 mg/day)	29.10/196.20[8]
	106.50/420.50[8]
5, 10, or 20 mg intranasally; can be repeated after 2 hrs (max 40 mg/day)	52.90/84.00[8]
22 mg intranasally; can be repeated after 2 hrs (max 44 g/day)	108.80
10 mg intranasally; can be repeated after 1 hr (max 30 mg/day)	97.50
3 mg SC; can be repeated after 1 hr (max 12 mg/day)	172.80
2.5 or 5 mg PO; can be repeated after 2 hrs (max 10 mg/day)[10]	13.40
	6.90
	129.40
	129.40
2.5 or 5 mg intranasally; can be repeated after 2 hrs (max 10 mg/day)[10]	89.00

6. Dose for pediatric patients is 5 mg (<40 kg) or 10 mg (≥40 kg). In pediatric patients, the efficacy and safety of redosing within 24 hours have not been established.
7. Adults and children (≥40 kg) also taking propranolol should use a 5-mg dose (max 15 mg/day for adults and 5 mg/day for children). Concurrent use of rizatriptan and propranolol is not recommended for children weighing <40 kg.
8. Cost of generic/cost of *Imitrex*.
9. Also available in refill cartridges for the auto-injectors, and generically as a 6-mg syringe.
10. Patients also taking cimetidine should use a 2.5-mg dose (max 5 mg/day).

Continued on next page

Table 2. Some Drugs for Acute Treatment of Migraine (continued)	
Drug	Some Formulations
Triptan/NSAID Combination	
Sumatriptan/naproxen[3] – generic Treximet (Curax)	10/60, 85/500 mg tabs
Calcitonin Gene-Related Peptide (GCRP) Receptor Antagonists	
Rimegepant – Nurtec ODT (Biohaven)	75 mg orally disintegrating tabs[12]
Ubrogepant – Ubrelvy (Allergan)	50, 100 mg tabs[13]
5-HT$_{1F}$ Receptor Agonist	
Lasmiditan[14] – Reyvow (Lilly)	50, 100 mg tabs
NSAIDs[15]	
Diclofenac potassium – Cambia (Assertio)	50 mg single-dose packets
Celecoxib – Elyxyb (Dr. Reddy's)	120 mg/4.8 mL oral solution
Ergots	
Dihydroergotamine mesylate – generic D.H.E. 45 (Bausch)	1 mg/mL ampules
generic Migranal nasal spray (Bausch)	4 mg/mL nasal spray
Ergotamine tartrate – Ergomar (TerSera)	2 mg sublingual tabs
Ergotamine/caffeine – generic Cafergot (Sandoz)	1/100 mg tabs
Migergot (Cosette)	2/100 mg rectal suppository

N.A. = cost not yet available
11. Dosage for adolescents 12-17 years old is 10/60 mg (max 85/500 mg/day).
12. Supplied in cartons containing a blister pack of 8 orally disintegrating tablets.

SELECTIVE 5-HT$_{1F}$ RECEPTOR AGONIST — Lasmiditan *(Reyvow)* selectively binds to 5-HT$_{1F}$ receptors expressed on trigeminal neurons, inhibiting pain pathways in the central and peripheral trigeminal system. In clinical trials, freedom from headache pain 2 hours post-dose occurred in a higher percentage of patients treated with lasmiditan (~30%) than with placebo (15-20%). Headache pain relief and freedom from the most bothersome migraine symptom also occurred more often with lasmiditan.[18] No

Usual Adult Dosage[1]	Cost[2]
85/500 mg PO; can be repeated after 2 hrs (max 170/1000 mg/day)[11]	$47.70
	129.80
75 mg PO (max 75 mg/day)	106.30
50 or 100 mg PO; can be repeated after 2 hrs (max 200 mg/day)	85.00
50, 100, or 200 mg PO (max 1 dose/day)	80.00
50 mg PO dissolved in 1-2 oz water once	83.10
120 mg PO once (max 1 dose/day)	N.A.
1 mg IM or SC; can be repeated at 1 hr intervals (max 3 mg/day, 6 mg/wk)	113.10
	1176.80
1 spray (0.5 mg) into each nostril, repeated 15 min later (2 mg/dose; max 3 mg/day, 4 mg/wk)	428.40
	477.90
2 mg SL; can be repeated at 30 min intervals (max 6 mg/day, 10 mg/wk)	61.40
2 tabs PO at attack onset, then 1 tab q30 min PRN (max 6 tabs/attack)	11.10
	12.30
1 suppository at attack onset, repeat in 1 hr if needed (max 2 suppositories/attack)	63.90

13. Supplied in boxes of 6, 8, 10, 12, or 30 unit-dose packets.
14. Classified as a schedule V controlled substance.
15. Other NSAIDs such as ibuprofen and naproxen are often used off-label.

trials directly comparing lasmiditan with triptans or with CGRP receptor antagonists are available.

Adverse Effects – Lasmiditan can cause CNS-related adverse effects including dizziness, paresthesia, sedation, vertigo, incoordination, cognitive changes, and confusion. Fatigue, nausea and vomiting, muscle weakness, lethargy, and palpitations have also been reported. Hypersensitivity reactions, including angioedema and rash, occurred in 0.2% of patients treated with lasmiditan in clinical trials. Increases in blood pressure, decreases in heart rate, and reactions consistent with serotonin syndrome have also been reported. Lasmiditan has not been shown to have vasoconstrictive effects.

In studies in healthy volunteers, single doses of lasmiditan have been found to decrease wakefulness and impair driving ability. The lasmiditan labeling warns against driving or operating machinery for at least 8 hours after taking the drug. Lasmiditan is classified as a schedule V controlled substance.

Drug Interactions – Use of lasmiditan with alcohol or other CNS depressants could result in additive effects. Coadministration of lasmiditan with serotonergic drugs might increase the risk of serotonin syndrome. Whether it is safe to use both lasmiditan and a triptan within a 24-hour period has not been determined. Lasmiditan should be used with caution in patients who are taking other heart rate-lowering drugs. Lasmiditan inhibits P-gp and BCRP; coadministration with P-gp or BCRP substrates should be avoided.

Pregnancy and Lactation – No data on the use of lasmiditan in pregnant or lactating women are available. Lasmiditan and its metabolites have been detected in the milk of lactating rats.

ERGOTS — A fixed-dose combination of **ergotamine tartrate**, a nonspecific serotonin agonist and vasoconstrictor, and caffeine is available in tablets *(Cafergot)* and suppositories *(Migergot)* for treatment of moderate to severe migraine. The combination is less effective than a triptan for acute treatment of migraine.[20]

Dihydroergotamine, which can be administered parenterally, can be effective in some patients whose migraine headaches do not respond to triptans. Dihydroergotamine nasal spray relieves migraine headache pain after 2 hours in about 50% of patients, with a 15% incidence of recurrence within 24 hours.[21]

Adverse Effects – Dihydroergotamine is a weaker arterial vasocon-strictor than ergotamine and causes fewer serious adverse effects. Nausea and vomiting are fairly common with ergotamine, but pretreatment with or concurrent use of an antiemetic such as metoclopramide can reduce GI adverse effects. Serious adverse effects, such as vascular (including coronary) occlusion and gangrene, are rare and are usually associated with overdosage (>6 mg in 24 hours or >10 mg per week). Hepatic impairment or fever can accelerate development of severe vasoconstric-tion. Ergots are contraindicated for use in patients with arterial disease or uncontrolled hypertension.

Drug Interactions – The effects of ergots can be potentiated by triptans, beta blockers, dopamine, nicotine. Concurrent use of ergots and strong CYP3A4 inhibitors is contraindicated.[12] Ergots and triptans should not be taken within 24 hours of each other.

Pregnancy and Lactation – Ergots can reduce placental blood flow and ergotamine is excreted in breast milk. Use of ergots in pregnant or breast-feeding women is contraindicated.

ANTIEMETICS — Parenteral formulations of the dopamine receptor antagonists **metoclopramide**, **prochlorperazine**, **chlorpromazine**, and **droperidol** can reduce nausea and headache pain in patients with migraine.[22] All of these drugs can cause extrapyramidal adverse effects. They can also prolong the QT interval, increasing the risk of torsades de pointes.

DEVICES — A **transcranial magnetic stimulation device** (*sTMS* – eNeura) is FDA-cleared for treatment of migraine in patients ≥12 years old. In one trial, the pain-free response rate 2 hours after treat-ment of the first migraine attack at the onset of aura was significantly higher with the device than with sham stimulation.[23]

A **remote electrical neuromodulation device** worn on the upper arm and controlled by a smartphone *(Nerivio)* is FDA-cleared for acute treatment of migraine in adults with <15 headache days/month. In a randomized, double-blind trial in 252 patients, it was significantly more effective than a sham device in relieving pain and the most bothersome migraine-associated symptom at 2 hours post-treatment.[24]

A **transcutaneous electrical nerve stimulation device** that is worn on the forehead *(Cefaly)* is FDA-cleared for acute treatment of migraine in adults. In a double-blind trial in 106 patients with acute migraine, use of the device for 1 hour was significantly more effective than sham treatment in reducing pain intensity.[25]

A portable **vagus nerve stimulation device** *(GammaCore)* is FDA-cleared for acute treatment of migraine-related pain in adults. In a randomized, double-blind trial in 248 patients, pain freedom occurred significantly more often with the active device than with a sham device at 30 and 60 minutes after initial use, but not at 120 minutes.[26]

MEDICATION OVERUSE HEADACHE — Overuse of drugs for acute treatment of migraine, particularly butalbital and opioids, can lead to chronic headache. Treatment of medication overuse headache involves withdrawing the overused drug(s); abrupt withdrawal may require hospitalization and bridge therapy with other drugs. Preventive treatment for migraine should be considered, and some expert clinicians suggest limiting future use of acute migraine treatments to ≤2 days per week.[27] CGRP receptor antagonists have not been associated with development of medication overuse headache.

PREVENTIVE TREATMENT OF MIGRAINE

Patients with migraine headaches that are frequent, severe, or refractory to acute treatment should receive preventive treatment.[1] Menstrual migraine headaches can sometimes be prevented by taking an NSAID or a triptan (particularly frovatriptan or naratriptan) for several days before and after the onset of menstruation.[28,29] Preventive therapy is generally not recommended during pregnancy.

BETA BLOCKERS — Beta blockers are commonly used for prevention of migraine. **Propranolol** and **timolol** are the only beta blockers that are FDA-approved for this indication, but **metoprolol, atenolol, bisoprolol**, and **nadolol** are also effective. Beta blockers can worsen asthma symptoms and cause fatigue, exercise intolerance, and orthostatic hypotension. They should not be used in patients with decompensated heart failure. Patients with migraine often have comorbid depression, which may be exacerbated by beta blockers.

ANTISEIZURE DRUGS — **Valproate** and **topiramate** are similarly effective in decreasing migraine frequency and are FDA-approved for migraine prevention. About 50% of patients achieve a ≥50% reduction in headache frequency with these drugs.[30] In randomized, double-blind trials, topiramate was at least as effective as propranolol for migraine prevention.[31,32] Topiramate has reduced migraine frequency and improved associated symptoms in patients with ≥15 headache days/month for ≥3 months and medication overuse headache.[33,34] In a trial in pediatric patients, however, topiramate was no more effective than placebo in preventing migraine.[35]

Adverse Effects – Valproate can cause nausea, fatigue, tremor, weight gain, and hair loss. Acute hepatic failure, pancreatitis, and hyperammonemia (in patients with urea cycle disorders) occur rarely. Polycystic ovary syndrome, hyperinsulinemia, lipid abnormalities, hirsutism, and menstrual disturbances have also been reported.

Topiramate commonly causes paresthesias; fatigue, language and cognitive impairment, taste perversion, weight loss, and nephrolithiasis can also occur. Topiramate can rarely cause narrow-angle glaucoma, oligohidrosis, and symptomatic metabolic acidosis.

Use of topiramate or valproate during pregnancy has been associated with congenital malformations.[36,37]

ANTIDEPRESSANTS — Amitriptyline is the only **tricyclic** antidepressant that has been shown to be effective for migraine prevention in clinical

Table 3. Some Drugs for Preventive Treatment of Migraine	
Drug	Some Formulations
Beta Blockers	
Metoprolol[3] – generic	25, 50, 100 mg tabs
Lopressor (Validus)	50, 100 mg tabs
extended-release – generic	25, 50, 100, 200 mg ER tabs
Toprol-XL (AstraZeneca)	
Propranolol – generic	10, 20, 40, 60, 80 mg tabs
extended-release – generic	60, 80, 120, 160 mg ER caps
Timolol – generic	5, 10, 20 mg tabs
Antiseizure Drugs	
Valproate[4] – generic	125, 250, 500 mg delayed-release
Depakote (Abbvie)	tabs; 125 mg sprinkle caps
extended-release – generic	250, 500 mg ER tabs
Depakote ER	
Topiramate[5] – generic	25, 50, 100, 200 mg tabs; 15,
Topamax (Janssen)	25 mg sprinkle caps
Calcitonin Gene-Related Peptide (CGRP) Antibodies[7]	
Eptinezumab-jjmr – *Vyepti* (Lundbeck)	100 mg/mL single-dose vials
Erenumab-aooe – *Aimovig* (Amgen/Novartis)	70, 140 mg/mL single-dose auto-injectors
Fremanezumab-vfrm – *Ajovy* (Teva)	225 mg/1.5 mL single-use syringes and auto-injectors
Galcanezumab-gnlm – *Emgality* (Lilly)	120 mg/1 mL single-use pens, syringes[10]
Tricyclic Antidepressants[3]	
Amitriptyline – generic	10, 25, 50, 75, 100, 150 mg tabs
Nortriptyline – generic	10, 25, 50, 75 mg caps

ER = extended-release
1. Dosage adjustments may be needed for renal or hepatic impairment or for drug interactions.
2. Approximate WAC for 30 days' treatment at the lowest usual dosage. The cost of eptinezumab is for one dose. WAC = wholesaler acquisition cost or manufacturer's published price to wholesalers; WAC represents a published catalogue or list price and may not represent an actual transactional price. Source: AnalySource® Monthly. September 5, 2020. Reprinted with permission by First Databank, Inc. All rights reserved. ©2020. www.fdbhealth.com/policies/drug-pricing-policy.
3. Not FDA-approved for this indication.
4. Oral formulations marketed as divalproex sodium (*Depakote*, and others) and valproic acid. Only divalproex sodium is FDA-approved for prevention of migraine. *Depakote Sprinkle Capsules* are not FDA-approved for prevention of migraine.

Usual Adult Dosage[1]	Cost[2]
50-100 mg PO bid	$3.20
	151.20
100-200 mg PO once/day	23.00
	59.20
40-160 mg PO divided bid	25.40
60-160 mg PO once/day	48.50
10-15 mg PO bid or 20 mg once/day	81.70
250-500 mg PO bid	12.00
	209.30
500-1000 mg PO once/day	34.80
	193.00
50 mg PO bid[6]	22.50
	739.50
100 mg IV q3 months[8]	1495.00
70 mg SC once/month[9]	603.20
225 mg SC once/month or 675 mg q3 months	402.10
240 mg SC once, then 120 mg once/month	603.60
25-150 mg PO once/day	8.90
25-150 mg PO once/day	9.40

5. Extended-release formulations of topiramate (*Trokendi XR*; *Qudexy XR*, and generic) are not FDA-approved for migraine prevention.
6. Dosage should be titrated to 100 mg/day over 4 weeks: week 1: 25 mg in the evening; week 2: 25 mg morning and evening; week 3: 25 mg morning and 50 mg evening; week 4: 50 mg morning and evening.
7. Eptinezumab, fremanezumab, and galcanezumab target CGRP. Erenumab targets the CGRP receptor.
8. Some patients may require a 300-mg dose.
9. Some patients may benefit from a dosage of 140 mg once/month administered as 2 consecutive 70-mg SC injections.
10. Also available in cartons of three 100 mg/mL syringes for treatment of episodic cluster headache.

Continued on next page

Table 3. Some Drugs for Preventive Treatment of Migraine (continued)	
Drug	**Some Formulations**
Serotonin-Norepinephrine Reuptake Inhibitor (SNRI)[3]	
Venlafaxine – generic	25, 37.5, 50, 75, 100 mg tabs
extended-release – generic	37.5, 75, 150 mg caps, tabs; 225 mg caps
Effexor XR (Pfizer)	37.5, 75, 150 mg caps
Botulinum Toxin Type A	
OnabotulinumtoxinA – *Botox* (Allergan)[11]	100, 200 unit vials

11. *Botox* is FDA-approved for prevention of headaches in adult patients with chronic migraine. *Botox Cosmetic* is not FDA-approved for migraine prevention.
12. Total dosage of 155 units is divided over 7 specific head/neck muscle areas (detailed information provided in package insert).

trials,[38] but it often causes sedation, dry mouth, and weight gain. Other tricyclics such as nortriptyline, which may have fewer adverse effects, are frequently used as alternatives in adults. In a trial in pediatric patients, amitriptyline was not more effective than placebo in preventing migraine.[35]

The **serotonin-norepinephrine reuptake inhibitors (SNRIs)** venlafaxine and duloxetine may also be effective in preventing migraine.[39,40] Adverse effects include nausea, vomiting, sweating, tachycardia, urinary retention, and blood pressure elevations.

CGRP ANTIBODIES — The long-acting CGRP antibodies erenumab *(Aimovig)*, fremanezumab *(Ajovy)*, galcanezumab *(Emgality)*, and eptinezumab *(Vyepti)* have reduced the number of migraine days by about 1-2 per month compared to placebo in double-blind trials in patients with episodic or chronic migraine.[41-43] They may be effective when other therapies have failed.[44-46] No head-to-head trials comparing them to each other or to other migraine-preventive drugs are available. Erenumab has been shown to be safe and effective in women with menstrual migraine.[47]

Adverse Effects – Injection-site reactions and constipation are the most common adverse effects of CGRP antibodies. Hypersensitivity reactions have been reported.[48] CGRP suppression could theoretically increase

Usual Adult Dosage[1]	Cost[2]
25-50 mg PO tid	$35.10
75-150 mg PO once/day	61.80
	465.00
155 units IM q12 weeks[12]	1202.00[13]

13. Cost of one 200-unit vial.

cardiovascular risk; patients with significant cardiovascular disease were excluded from clinical trials. Use of these drugs has been associated with hypertension.

Pregnancy – No adequate data are available on use of CGRP antibodies in pregnant women. Because of their long half-lives, fetal exposure could occur for months after stopping these drugs.

OTHER PREVENTIVE DRUGS — Pericranial intramuscular injections of **onabotulinumtoxinA** *(Botox)* are FDA-approved for prevention of headache in adults with ≥15 migraine headaches/month.[49] Botulinum toxin is not recommended for prevention of episodic migraine.

NSAIDs, such as naproxen and ibuprofen, have been used for prevention of episodic migraine.[50] The antihypertensive drugs **lisinopril**, **candesartan**, and **verapamil** have reduced migraine frequency in some small studies.[51-53] The combination of **simvastatin** and **vitamin D** was effective for migraine prevention in one small, randomized, placebo-controlled trial.[54]

DEVICES — The *Cefaly* **transcutaneous electrical nerve stimulation device** is FDA-cleared for prevention of episodic migraine in adults. In one small trial, daily 20-minute treatments for 3 months were modestly effective in reducing migraine frequency.[55]

The *sTMS* **transcranial magnetic stimulation device** is FDA-cleared for prevention of migraine in patients ≥12 years old. In a prospective observational study, 12 weeks of preventive and as-needed treatment with the device reduced headache frequency compared to historical controls.[56]

The *GammaCore* **vagus nerve stimulation device** is FDA-cleared for prevention of migraine in adults. In a post-hoc analysis of a double-blind trial, use of the device for 4 minutes 3 times daily was associated with a reduction in migraine days, compared to use of a sham device, among patients with ≥67% adherence to the treatment regimen.[57]

ACUPUNCTURE — Many comparative studies have examined the efficacy of acupuncture for preventive treatment of migraine headaches.[58,59] It has been compared with no treatment, pharmacologic treatment, and sham treatment in studies of varying size and quality and has usually been found to be superior to no treatment, sometimes superior to pharmacologic treatment, and occasionally superior to sham treatment. Reviewers generally agree that acupuncture has a strong placebo effect and is associated with fewer adverse effects than pharmacotherapy.

1. American Headache Society. The American Headache Society position statement on integrating new migraine treatments into clinical practice. Headache 2019; 59:1.
2. M Oskoui et al. Practice guideline update summary: acute treatment of migraine in children and adolescents: report of the guideline development, dissemination, and implementation subcommittee of the American Academy of Neurology and the American Headache Society. Neurology 2019; 93:487.
3. MJ Prior et al. A randomized, placebo-controlled trial of acetaminophen for treatment of migraine headache. Headache 2010; 50:819.
4. CC Suthisisang et al. Meta-analysis of the efficacy and safety of naproxen sodium in the acute treatment of migraine. Headache 2010; 50:808.
5. C Suthisisang et al. Efficacy of low-dose ibuprofen in acute migraine treatment: systematic review and meta-analysis. Ann Pharmacother 2007; 41:1782.
6. C Chen et al. Differential pharmacokinetics of diclofenac potassium for oral solution vs immediate-release tablets from a randomized trial: effect of fed and fasting conditions. Headache 2015; 55:265.

7. MM Johnston and AM Rapoport. Triptans for the management of migraine. Drugs 2010; 70:1505.
8. Onzetra Xsail - sumatriptan nasal powder. Med Lett Drugs Ther 2016; 58:92.
9. CJ Derry et al. Sumatriptan (all routes of administration) for acute migraine attacks in adults – overview of Cochrane reviews. Cochrane Database Syst Rev 2014; 5:CD009108.
10. S Law et al. Sumatriptan plus naproxen for the treatment of acute migraine attacks in adults. Cochrane Database Syst Rev 2016; 4:CD008541.
11. G Roberto et al. Triptans and serious adverse vascular events: data mining of the FDA Adverse Event Reporting System database. Cephalalgia 2014; 34:5.
12. Inhibitors and inducers of CYP enzymes and P-glycoprotein. Med Lett Drugs Ther 2020 September 10 (epub). Available at: http://secure.medicalletter.org/downloads/CYP_PGP_ Tables.pdf.
13. RG Wenzel et al. Serotonin syndrome risks when combining SSRI/SNRI drugs with triptans: is the FDA's alert warranted? Ann Pharmacother 2008; 42:1692.
14. Y Orlova et al. Association of coprescription of triptan antimigraine drugs and selective serotonin reuptake inhibitor or selective norepinephrine reuptake inhibitor antidepressants with serotonin syndrome. JAMA Neurol 2018; 75:566.
15. K Nezvalová-Henriksen et al. Triptan safety during pregnancy: a Norwegian population registry study. Eur J Epidemiol 2013; 28:759.
16. US National Library of Medicine. Drugs and Lactation Data-base (LactMed). Available at: www.ncbi.nlm.nih.gov/books/NBK501922/. Accessed September 24, 2020.
17. AD Hershey. CGRP – the next frontier for migraine. N Engl J Med 2017; 377:2190.
18. Lasmiditan (Reyvow) and ubrogepant (Ubrelvy) for acute treatment of migraine. Med Lett Drugs Ther 2020; 62:35.
19. Rimegepant (Nurtec ODT) for acute treatment of migraine. Med Lett Drugs Ther 2020; 62:70.
20. MJA Láinez et al. Crossover, double-blind clinical trial comparing almotriptan and ergotamine plus caffeine for acute migraine therapy. Eur J Neurol 2007; 14:269.
21. SD Silberstein et al. Dihydroergotamine (DHE) – then and now: a narrative review. Headache 2020; 60:40.
22. MJ Marmura et al. The acute treatment of migraine in adults: the American Headache Society evidence assessment of migraine pharmacotherapies. Headache 2015; 55:3.
23. RB Lipton et al. Single-pulse transcranial magnetic stimulation for acute treatment of migraine with aura: a randomised, double-blind, parallel-group, sham-controlled trial. Lancet Neurol 2010; 9:373.
24. D Yarnitsky et al. Remote electrical neuromodulation (REN) relieves acute migraine: a randomized, double-blind, placebo-controlled, multicenter trial. Headache 2019; 59:1240.
25. DE Chou et al. Acute migraine therapy with external trigeminal neurostimulation (ACME): a randomized controlled trial. Cephalalgia 2019; 39:3.
26. C Tassorelli et al. Noninvasive vagus nerve stimulation as acute therapy for migraine: the randomized PRESTO study. Neurology 2018; 91:e364.
27. JR Saper and AN Da Silva. Medication overuse headache: history, features, prevention and management strategies. CNS Drugs 2013; 27:867.
28. T Pringsheim et al. Acute treatment and prevention of menstrually related migraine headache: evidence-based review. Neurology 2008; 70:1555.

29. EA MacGregor et al. Safety and tolerability of frovatriptan in the acute treatment of migraine and prevention of menstrual migraine: results of a new analysis of data from five previously published studies. Gend Med 2010; 7:88.
30. WM Mulleners et al. Antiepileptics in migraine prophylaxis: an updated Cochrane review. Cephalalgia 2015; 35:51.
31. H-C Diener et al. Topiramate in migraine prophylaxis–results from a placebo-controlled trial with propranolol as an active control. J Neurol 2004; 251:943.
32. F Ashtari et al. A double-blind, randomized trial of low-dose topiramate vs propranolol in migraine prophylaxis. Acta Neurol Scand 2008; 118:301.
33. S Silberstein et al. Topiramate treatment of chronic migraine: a randomized, placebo-controlled trial of quality of life and other efficacy measures. Headache 2009; 49:1153.
34. H-C Diener et al. Topiramate reduces headache days in chronic migraine: a randomized, double-blind, placebo-controlled study. Cephalalgia 2007; 27:814.
35. SW Powers et al. Trial of amitriptyline, topiramate, and placebo for pediatric migraine. N Engl J Med 2017; 376:115.
36. In brief: Warning against use of valproate for migraine prevention during pregnancy. Med Lett Drugs Ther 2013; 55:45.
37. J Weston et al. Monotherapy treatment of epilepsy in pregnancy: congenital malformation outcomes in the child. Cochrane Database Syst Rev 2016; 11:CD010224.
38. DW Dodick et al. Topiramate versus amitriptyline in migraine prevention: a 26-week, multicenter, randomized, double-blind, double-dummy, parallel-group noninferiority trial in adult migraineurs. Clin Ther 2009; 31:542.
39. S Tarlaci. Escitalopram and venlafaxine for the prophylaxis of migraine headache without mood disorders. Clin Neuropharmacol 2009; 32:254.
40. WB Young et al. Duloxetine prophylaxis for episodic migraine in persons without depression: a prospective study. Headache 2013; 53:1430.
41. Erenumab (Aimovig) for migraine prevention. Med Lett Drugs Ther 2018; 60:101.
42. Fremanezumab (Ajovy) and galcanezumab (Emgality) for migraine prevention. Med Lett Drugs Ther 2018; 60:177.
43. Eptinezumab (Vyepti) for migraine prevention. Med Lett Drugs Ther 2020; 62:85.
44. A Scheffler et al. Erenumab in highly therapy-refractory migraine patients: first German real-world evidence. J Headache Pain 2020; 21:84.
45. MD Ferrari et al. Fremanezumab versus placebo for migraine prevention in patients with documented failure to up to four migraine preventive medication classes (FOCUS): a randomised, double-blind, placebo-controlled, phase 3b trial. Lancet 2019; 394:1030.
46. WM Mulleners et al. Safety and efficacy of galcanezumab in patients for whom previous migraine preventive medication from two to four categories had failed (CONQUER): a multicentre, randomised, double-blind, placebo-controlled, phase 3b trial. Lancet Neurol 2020; 19:814.
47. JM Pavlovic et al. Efficacy and safety of erenumab in women with a history of menstrual migraine. J Headache Pain 2020; 21:95.
48. In brief: Erenumab (Aimovig) hypersensitivity. Med Lett Drugs Ther 2019; 61:48.
49. Botulinum toxin for chronic migraine. Med Lett Drugs Ther 2011; 53:7.
50. S Holland et al. Evidence-based guideline update: NSAIDs and other complementary treatments for episodic migraine prevention in adults: report of the Quality Standards

Subcommittee of the American Academy of Neurology and the American Headache Society. Neurology 2012; 78:1346.

51. BJ Gales et al. Angiotensin-converting enzyme inhibitors and angiotensin receptor blockers for the prevention of migraines. Ann Pharmacother 2010; 44:360.

52. LJ Stovner et al. A comparative study of candesartan versus propranolol for migraine prophylaxis: a randomised, triple-blind, placebo-controlled, double cross-over study. Cephalalgia 2014; 34:523.

53. JL Jackson et al. A comparative effectiveness meta-analysis of drugs for the prophylaxis of migraine headache. PLoS One 2015; 10:e0130733.

54. C Buettner et al. Simvastatin and vitamin D for migraine prevention: a randomized, controlled trial. Ann Neurol 2015; 78:970.

55. A transcutaneous electrical nerve stimulation device (Cefaly) for migraine prevention. Med Lett Drugs Ther 2014; 56:78.

56. AJ Starling et al. A multicenter, prospective, single arm, open label, observational study of sTMS for migraine prevention (ESPOUSE Study). Cephalalgia 2018; 38:1038.

57. H-C Diener et al. Non-invasive vagus nerve stimulation (nVNS) for the preventive treatment of episodic migraine: the multicentre, double-blind, randomised, sham-controlled PREMIUM trial. Cephalalgia 2019; 39:1475.

58. X Ni et al. Acupuncture versus various control treatments in the treatment of migraine: a review of randomized controlled trials from the past 10 years. J Pain Res 2020; 13:2033.

59. S-Q Fan et al. Efficacy of acupuncture for migraine prophylaxis: a trial sequential meta-analysis. J Neurol 2020 Aug 24 (epub).

DRUGS FOR
Osteoarthritis

Original publication date — April 2020 (revised October 2020)

Many different drugs are used for treatment of osteoarthritis pain, but none of them prevent progression of the disease. Nonpharmacologic approaches including weight management, exercise, tai chi, physical therapy, assistive devices, and total joint arthroplasty can also be used. The American College of Rheumatology (ACR) has published new guidelines for the management of osteoarthritis of the hip, hand, and knee.[1]

NSAIDS

Nonsteroidal anti-inflammatory drugs (NSAIDs) are preferred for initial treatment of osteoarthritis pain in patients without risk factors for serious adverse effects; they should be used at the lowest effective dose, especially in older adults.[2] If one NSAID is ineffective, switching to another may provide better pain control. Topical NSAIDs should be considered before oral NSAIDs for treatment of knee or hand osteoarthritis pain; they appear to be similar in efficacy and have a lower risk of systemic adverse effects.[3]

BLEEDING — All NSAIDs except salsalate and COX-2 selective celecoxib (*Celebrex*, and generics) can interfere with platelet function and prolong bleeding time. Unlike aspirin, which irreversibly inhibits platelet activity for the life of the platelet (up to 10 days), NSAID-induced antiplatelet effects are reversed when the NSAID is cleared.

Summary: Drugs for Osteoarthritis

▶ NSAIDs are effective for treatment of osteoarthritis pain, but they can cause serious GI, renal, and cardiovascular toxicity, especially in older adults.

▶ Topical NSAIDs should be considered before oral NSAIDs for treatment of knee or hand osteoarthritis pain.

▶ COX-2 selective celecoxib does not interfere with platelet function and is less likely than nonselective NSAIDs to cause GI toxicity. It may have a prothrombotic effect, but in the dosage recommended for treatment of osteoarthritis (200 mg/day), its cardiovascular safety appears to be comparable to that of naproxen and ibuprofen.

▶ Acetaminophen is less effective than NSAIDs, but in doses ≤4 g/day it generally causes fewer adverse effects. In higher doses, it can cause severe hepatotoxicity. Acetaminophen can be tried when topical and oral NSAIDs are not recommended or poorly tolerated.

▶ The serotonin and norepinephrine reuptake inhibitor duloxetine is another alternative. It is only modestly effective and has many adverse effects.

▶ Opioids appear to be only moderately more effective than placebo for treatment of osteoarthritis pain, and their continued use can lead to dependence and development of tolerance to their effects. They should be considered a last resort for patients with intractable osteoarthritis pain.

▶ Intra-articular corticosteroid injections are generally safe and effective for local treatment of osteoarthritis. Pain relief tends to wane by 2 months after administration, but most clinicians wait at least 3 months between injections.

GASTROINTESTINAL TOXICITY — Dyspepsia and GI ulceration, perforation, and bleeding can occur with all NSAIDs, including parenteral formulations. Serious GI complications can occur without warning. High doses, prolonged use, previous peptic ulcer disease, excessive alcohol intake, smoking, advanced age, and concomitant use of systemic corticosteroids, aspirin (even 81 mg/day), warfarin, or other anticoagulants increase the risk of these complications. Concurrent use of a proton pump inhibitor, an H_2-receptor antagonist, or the prostaglandin analog misoprostol (*Cytotec*, and generics) may decrease the incidence of NSAID-induced GI toxicity. Celecoxib is less likely than nonselective NSAIDs to cause GI toxicity.[4] Diclofenac, etodolac, meloxicam, and nabumetone are somewhat COX-2 selective *in vitro*. Theoretically, these drugs could cause less GI toxicity than less selective NSAIDs such as ibuprofen, but there are no clinical data showing that they are less likely to cause serious GI complications, and only weak data suggesting that they are less likely to cause symptomatic ulcers.

RENAL TOXICITY — All NSAIDs, including celecoxib, inhibit renal prostaglandins, decrease renal blood flow, and increase fluid retention. They can cause hypertension and renal failure, particularly in the elderly. Diminished renal function or decreased effective intravascular volume due to diuretic therapy, cirrhosis, or heart failure increases the risk of NSAID-induced renal toxicity.

CARDIOVASCULAR EFFECTS — NSAIDs, especially COX-2 selective NSAIDs, may have a prothrombotic effect and have been associated with an increased risk of serious cardiovascular events, including myocardial infarction, stroke, and pulmonary edema.[5]

In the PRECISION trial, 24,081 patients with osteoarthritis (90%) or rheumatoid arthritis (10%) and established cardiovascular disease or elevated cardiovascular risk were randomized to receive COX-2 selective celecoxib 100 mg twice daily, ibuprofen 600 mg three times daily, or naproxen 375 mg twice daily; the mean treatment duration was 20.3 months and the mean follow-up period was 34.1 months. A primary outcome event (cardiovascular death, nonfatal myocardial infarction, or nonfatal stroke) occurred in 2.3% of patients taking celecoxib, 2.5% taking naproxen, and 2.7% taking ibuprofen; celecoxib was determined to be noninferior to both ibuprofen and naproxen with respect to cardiovascular safety.[6] This trial had significant limitations; notably, increases were permitted in the dosages of ibuprofen and naproxen, but not in the dosage of celecoxib (200 mg/day is the maximum recommended dose of celecoxib for treatment of osteoarthritis). Also, by the end of the trial, 69% of the patients had stopped taking their assigned drug.[7]

OTHER ADVERSE EFFECTS — NSAIDs can precipitate asthma and anaphylactoid reactions in aspirin-sensitive patients. They frequently cause small increases in aminotransferase activity. Serious hepatotoxicity

Table 1. Some Systemic Analgesics for Osteoarthritis

Drug	Some Formulations
Acetaminophen – generic *Tylenol* (McNeil Consumer)	325, 500 mg tabs; 650 mg ER tabs[3]
Some Nonselective NSAIDs	

Diclofenac – *Zorvolex* (Zyla)
Diclofenac potassium – generic
Diclofenac sodium – generic
  extended-release – generic
  Voltaren-XR (Novartis)
	18, 35 mg caps
	50 mg tabs
	25, 50, 75 mg DR tabs
	100 mg ER tabs

Etodolac – generic extended-release – generic	200, 300 mg caps; 400, 500 mg tabs 400, 500, 600 mg ER tabs
Fenoprofen – generic *Nalfon* (Xspire)	400 mg caps; 600 mg tabs 400 mg caps
Flurbiprofen – generic	50, 100 mg tabs
Ibuprofen – generic *Advil* (Pfizer)	200, 400, 600, 800 mg tabs; 200 mg caps[3]
Ketoprofen – generic extended-release – generic	50, 75 mg caps 200 mg ER caps
Meclofenamate – generic	50, 100 mg caps

Meloxicam – generic
  Mobic (Boehringer Ingelheim)
  Vivlodex (Zyla)
	7.5, 15 mg tabs
	
	5, 10 mg caps

Nabumetone – generic	500, 750 mg tabs

Naproxen[6] – generic
  Naprosyn, EC-Naprosyn (Genentech)
Naproxen sodium – generic
  Anaprox DS (Genentech)
Naproxen sodium OTC – generic
  Aleve (Bayer)
	250, 375, 500 mg tabs; 375, 500 mg
	  enteric-coated tabs; 25 mg/mL PO susp[7]
	275, 550 mg tabs
	550 mg tabs
	220 mg tabs, caps

Salsalate – generic	500, 750 mg tabs

DR = delayed-release; ER = extended-release
1. Usual dosage for treatment of osteoarthritis. Dosage adjustments may be needed for hepatic or renal impairment. NSAIDs, acetaminophen, and tramadol should be taken on an as-needed basis.
2. Approximate WAC for 30 days' treatment with the lowest usual dosage using the smallest possible number of whole dosage units. WAC = wholesaler acquisition cost or manufacturer's published price to wholesalers; WAC represents a published catalogue or list price and may not represent an actual transactional price. Source: AnalySource® Monthly. April 5, 2020. Reprinted with permission by First Databank, Inc. All rights reserved. ©2020. www.fdbhealth.com/drug-pricing-policy.
3. Available in multiple strengths and dosage forms, alone and in combination with other drugs, both over the counter and by prescription.

Usual Dosage[1]	Max Daily Dose	Cost[2]
650 mg qid or 1000 mg tid	4000 mg	$4.60
		11.60
35 mg tid	105 mg	714.40
50 mg bid or tid	200 mg[4]	62.70
100-150 mg divided bid or tid	150 mg	15.90
100 mg once/day	200 mg[5]	67.50
		309.90
300 mg bid or tid or 400-500 mg bid	1000 mg	22.50
400-1000 mg once/day	1000 mg	56.90
400-600 mg tid or qid	3200 mg	335.10
		467.80
200-300 mg divided bid-qid	300 mg (100 mg/dose)	25.20
200-400 mg q4-6h	3200 mg (1200 mg OTC)	6.50
		8.20
50 mg qid or 75 mg tid	300 mg	85.50
200 mg once/day	200 mg	259.60
50-100 mg qid	400 mg	400.20
7.5-15 mg once/day	15 mg	7.90
		268.40
5-10 mg once/day	10 mg	862.60
500-750 mg bid or tid	2000 mg	29.50
250-500 mg bid	1000 mg[8]	7.40
		133.00
275-550 mg bid	1100 mg[8]	62.50
		558.60
220 mg bid or tid	660 mg	2.60
		6.80
1500 mg bid or 1000 mg tid	3000 mg	95.60

4. The maximum recommended daily dose for treatment of osteoarthritis is 150 mg.
5. The maximum recommended daily dose for treatment of osteoarthritis is 100 mg.
6. Naproxen is also available in a fixed-dose combination with the proton pump inhibitor esomeprazole magnesium as *Vimovo*.
7. The suspension is not available generically. *Naprosyn* is not available in 250- or 375-mg tabs.
8. In patients who tolerate lower doses, the daily dose of naproxen may be increased to 1500 mg (1650 mg naproxen sodium) for periods of up to 6 months when additional anti-inflammatory or analgesic activity is required.

Continued on next page

Table 1. Some Systemic Analgesics for Osteoarthritis (continued)	
Drug	**Some Formulations**
Selective COX-2 Inhibitor	
Celecoxib – generic *Celebrex* (Pfizer)	50, 100, 200, 400 mg caps
Serotonin and Norepinephrine Reuptake Inhibitor	
Duloxetine – generic *Cymbalta* (Lilly)	20, 30, 60 mg delayed-release caps
Opioid Agonist/Serotonin and Norepinephrine Reuptake Inhibitor	
Tramadol[12] – generic *Ultram* (Janssen) extended-release tabs – generic extended-release caps – generic *Conzip* (Vertical)	50, 100 mg tabs 50 mg tabs 100, 200, 300 mg ER tabs 100, 150, 200, 300 mg ER caps 100, 200, 300 mg ER caps

DR = delayed-release; ER = extended-release
9. The initial dose should be reduced by 50% in patients who are CYP2C9 poor metabolizers.
10. The maximum recommended daily dose for treatment of osteoarthritis is 200 mg.

is rare, but may occur more frequently with diclofenac; transaminase levels should be monitored with regular use of all formulations of the drug, including the over-the-counter topical gel.[8] Cholestatic hepatitis has occurred with use of celecoxib. Pancreatitis has been reported with several NSAIDs.

NSAIDs can cause CNS adverse effects such as dizziness, anxiety, drowsiness, confusion, depression, disorientation, severe headache, and aseptic meningitis. They have been associated with both mild and severe skin reactions, including exfoliative dermatitis, Stevens-Johnson syndrome, and toxic epidermal necrolysis. NSAIDs rarely cause blood dyscrasias, including aplastic anemia.

PREGNANCY — Exposure to NSAIDs around the time of conception or during pregnancy has been associated with an increased risk of miscarriage, but the data are weak.[9] Use of NSAIDs during the third trimester

Usual Dosage[1]	Max Daily Dose	Cost[2]
200 mg once/day or 100 mg bid[9]	400 mg[10]	$51.50
		398.40
30 mg once/day for 7 days, then 60 mg once/day	120 mg[11]	21.40
		256.80
50-100 mg q4-6 hrs	400 mg	10.00
		410.40
100-300 mg once/day	300 mg	63.30
100-300 mg once/day	300 mg	229.60
		341.80

11. The maximum recommended daily dose for treatment of osteoarthritis is 60 mg.
12. Not FDA-approved for treatment of osteoarthritis. Tramadol is also available in a fixed-dose combination with acetaminophen (*Ultracet*, and generics).

of pregnancy may cause premature closure of the ductus arteriosus and persistent pulmonary hypertension in the neonate, but these effects appear to be uncommon if the drug is stopped 6-8 weeks before delivery.

DRUG INTERACTIONS — NSAIDs may decrease the effectiveness of diuretics, beta blockers, ACE inhibitors, and some other antihypertensive drugs, and can increase serum concentrations and the toxicity of lithium and methotrexate. Concomitant use of NSAIDs with warfarin or other anticoagulants is generally discouraged. Patients taking aspirin for cardiovascular protection should not take NSAIDs regularly because, except for celecoxib, they can interfere with the antiplatelet effect of aspirin. Celecoxib is a moderate CYP2D6 inhibitor; it can increase serum concentrations of CYP2D6 substrates. Celecoxib, diclofenac, flurbiprofen, ibuprofen, indomethacin, meloxicam, naproxen, and piroxicam are CYP2C9 substrates; dosage reductions may be required in CYP2C9 poor metabolizers and patients taking a CYP2C9 inhibitor.[10]

Table 2. Some Topical Analgesics for Osteoarthritis

Drug	Some Formulations
Capsaicin[2] — *Capzasin-HP* (Chattem)	0.1% cream (42.5 g)
Aspercreme Warming (Chattem)	0.025% patches (5 ct)
Diclofenac epolamine[4] — generic	1.3% patch (30 ct)
Flector (Pfizer)	
Diclofenac sodium solution[5] — generic	1.5% topical soln (150 mL)
Pennsaid (Mallinckrodt)	2% topical soln (112 g)
gel — generic	1% gel (100 g)
Voltaren Arthritis Pain[6] (GSK)	

1. Approximate WAC for the listed package size. WAC = wholesaler acquisition cost or manufacturer's published price to wholesalers; WAC represents a published catalogue or list price and may not represent an actual transactional price. Source: AnalySource® Monthly. April 5, 2020. Reprinted with permission by First Databank, Inc. All rights reserved. ©2020. www.fdbhealth.com/drug-pricing-policy.
2. Available over the counter. Also available in other brands and dosage forms.
3. Cost according to cvs.com. Accessed April 9, 2020.
4. Not FDA-approved for treatment of osteoarthritis.

ACETAMINOPHEN

Acetaminophen has fewer adverse effects than NSAIDs, but it has no clinically significant anti-inflammatory activity and is less effective for treatment of osteoarthritis. In a large meta-analysis, acetaminophen monotherapy at doses up to 3000 mg/day was not found to be significantly more effective than placebo in reducing hip or knee osteoarthritis pain.[11] Acetaminophen can be tried in doses up to 4000 mg/day when topical and oral NSAID treatment are not recommended or are poorly tolerated.

ADVERSE EFFECTS — Most healthy patients can take up to 4 grams of acetaminophen daily with no adverse effects. A dosage of 1 gram three times daily for 2 weeks has been shown to increase blood pressure in patients with cardiovascular disease.[12] Acetaminophen overdose can cause serious or fatal hepatotoxicity. In some patients, such as those who are fasting, are heavy alcohol users, or are concurrently taking isoniazid (INH), zidovudine (*Retrovir*, and generics), or a barbiturate, hepatotoxicity can develop after moderate overdosage or even with high therapeutic doses (3-4 g/day). Regular monitoring of liver function is recommended

Usual Dosage	Cost[1]
Apply tid or qid	$17.99[3]
Apply up to tid (max 8 hrs/patch)	9.99[3]
1 patch bid	273.00
	373.00
40 drops per knee qid	643.90
40 mg (2 pump actuations) per knee bid	2487.40
2-4 g qid[7] (max 32 g/day)[8]	35.30
	54.00

5. FDA-approved only for knee osteoarthritis.
6. Expected to become available over-the-counter in spring 2020; will no longer be available by prescription.
7. The dose for lower extremities is 4 g and for upper extremities is 2 g.
8. The maximum dose is 16 g/day applied to any one joint of the lower extremities and 8 g/day applied to any one joint of the upper extremities.

for all patients who take high doses of acetaminophen. Continued use of acetaminophen may increase the anticoagulant effect of warfarin in some patients.[13] Some meta-analyses of cohort and case-control studies have suggested that long-term use of the drug may increase the risk of renal cell cancer.[14]

PREGNANCY — Acetaminophen causes fetal toxicity in animals; no controlled trials of its use in pregnant women are available. Occasional use of oral acetaminophen during pregnancy is generally considered safe, but some reports have associated its use in pregnant women with an increased risk of attention-deficit/hyperactivity disorder (ADHD) and autism spectrum disorder in children.[15,16]

DULOXETINE

The serotonin and norepinephrine reuptake inhibitor (SNRI) duloxetine (*Cymbalta*, and generics) is FDA-approved for treatment of chronic musculoskeletal pain.[17] It appears to be effective for treatment of osteoarthritis pain both alone and as an adjunct to NSAID treatment, but its

Table 3. Some Intra-Articular Corticosteroids for Osteoarthritis	
Drug	Some Formulations
Methylprednisolone acetate – generic	40, 80 mg/mL vials
Depo-Medrol (Pfizer)	20, 40, 80 mg/mL vials
Triamcinolone acetonide – generic	40 mg/mL vials
Kenalog (BMS)	10, 40 mg/mL vials
extended-release – *Zilretta*[4] (Flexion)	32 mg powder for reconstitution

1. Approximate WAC for one unit of the lowest-strength formulation. WAC = wholesaler acquisition cost or manufacturer's published price to wholesalers; WAC represents a published catalogue or list price and may not represent an actual transactional price. Source: AnalySource® Monthly. April 5, 2020. Reprinted with permission by First Databank, Inc. All rights reserved. ©2020. www.fdbhealth.com/drug-pricing-policy.

effect size in clinical trials has been modest and its long-term efficacy for this indication is unknown.[18] Duloxetine can cause headache, nausea, somnolence, insomnia, dry mouth, constipation, diarrhea, decreased appetite, hyperhidrosis, and blood pressure elevations. Serious, sometimes fatal, hepatotoxicity, serotonin syndrome, severe skin reactions, orthostatic hypotension, and syncope can occur. Like other drugs that inhibit reuptake of serotonin, duloxetine can increase the risk of bleeding.

Duloxetine is a substrate of CYP1A2 and CYP2D6; coadministration of strong CYP1A2 inhibitors such as ciprofloxacin should be avoided, and dosage reductions may be needed with coadministration of strong CYP2D6 inhibitors such as terbinafine and in CYP2D6 poor metabolizers. Duloxetine itself is a moderate CYP2D6 inhibitor; it can increase serum concentrations of other CYP2D6 substrates.[10]

OPIOIDS

Long-term use of opioid agonists to treat chronic noncancer pain is problematic and its benefits are questionable. In a meta-analysis of 96 trials in patients with chronic noncancer pain, opioids modestly reduced pain compared to placebo, and their effectiveness decreased over time.[19] Opioids can be tried as a last resort for treatment of intractable osteoarthritis pain; they should be used at the lowest effective dose for the

Usual Dosage[2]	Cost[1]
4-10 mg once (small joints); 10-40 mg once (medium joints);	$7.30
20-80 mg once (large joints)	33.10
2.5-10 mg once (small joints); 5-40 mg once (large joints)[3]	8.30
	9.40
32 mg once[5]	570.00

2. Pain relief usually lasts for at least one month; by 2 months, the effect tends to wane. Most clinicians wait a minimum of 3 months between injections.
3. Maximum of 80 mg per single treatment period.
4. FDA-approved only for treatment of knee osteoarthritis.
5. Not FDA-approved for repeat administration.

shortest possible duration.[20] With continued use, patients become tolerant to both their analgesic and adverse effects, except for constipation.

TRAMADOL — A weak opioid agonist that also inhibits reuptake of serotonin and norepinephrine, tramadol (*Ultram*, and others) is FDA-approved for treatment of adults with pain severe enough to require an opioid and for which alternative treatments are inadequate.[21] In clinical trials, extended-release tramadol was modestly more effective than placebo in reducing moderate to severe osteoarthritis knee pain, but a substantial number of patients discontinued it because of adverse effects including nausea, vomiting, constipation, dizziness, and somnolence. Hypoglycemia can also occur. Seizures have been reported with use of tramadol; patients with a history of seizures and those concomitantly taking a tricyclic antidepressant, a serotonin reuptake inhibitor, a monoamine oxidase (MAO) inhibitor, other opioids, or an antipsychotic drug may be at increased risk. Tramadol is classified as a schedule IV controlled substance because it can cause psychological and physical dependence.

Tramadol is demethylated by CYP2D6 to a metabolite (M1) that has more potent opioid activity than tramadol itself; CYP2D6 poor metabolizers and patients taking CYP2D6 inhibitors (such as celecoxib) may experience decreased analgesic effects and opioid withdrawal symptoms. Concurrent use of tramadol with drugs that inhibit CYP2D6 or 3A4 can also increase tramadol levels and the risk of seizures and serotonin syndrome.[10] CYP2D6 ultra-rapid metabolizers may be at risk for serious opioid adverse effects, including respiratory depression.

Tramadol is conditionally recommended by the ACR over other opioids for treatment of osteoarthritis, but its unpredictable pharmacokinetics and potential for serious adverse drug interactions have led some Medical Letter reviewers to advise against its use.

DIETARY SUPPLEMENTS

Glucosamine stimulates cartilage cells *in vitro* to synthesize glycos-aminoglycans and proteoglycans. When given orally to animals, it has a modest anti-inflammatory effect. The glycosaminoglycan **chondroitin sulfate** has been reported in animals to maintain viscosity in joints, stim-ulate cartilage repair mechanisms, and inhibit enzymes that break down cartilage. The effectiveness of these agents in humans remains to be estab-lished. Neither glucosamine nor chondroitin sulfate is FDA-approved for any indication, but both are widely available as dietary supplements and heavily promoted for "management of joint health."

The ACR strongly recommends against use of glucosamine because the weight of the evidence indicates a lack of efficacy and large placebo effects. It also recommends against use of chondroitin for treatment of knee or hip osteoarthritis, but conditionally recommends its use for treatment of hand osteoarthritis based on the results of one 6-month double-blind trial in 162 patients, in which chondroitin sulfate 800 mg once/day was modestly more effective than placebo in improving pain and hand function.[22] Chondroitin and glucosamine appear to be safe, but as with other dietary supplements, the potency and purity of the products may vary.

Turmeric is also widely promoted for pain relief and joint mobility. No large randomized controlled trials evaluating its effectiveness are available, but in one 12-week, double-blind trial in 70 patients, turmeric 1000 mg/day reduced knee osteoarthritis pain significantly more than placebo.[30] Turmeric has not been approved by the FDA for any indication.[23]

CAPSAICIN

The vanillyl alkaloid capsaicin, which is found in hot peppers and related plants, is available over the counter in various brands and has been used topically to treat osteoarthritis. It appears to reduce knee osteoarthritis pain in some patients,[24] but it can cause severe skin burns and nerve damage at the application site, and the dried residue can cause coughing, sneezing, and eye irritation.[25] Because of the risk of eye contamination, capsaicin is not recommended for treatment of hand osteoarthritis pain.

INTRA-ARTICULAR INJECTIONS

Many patients with osteoarthritis have inadequate responses or relative contraindications to systemic anti-inflammatory or analgesic drugs. Injectable intra-articular agents, particularly corticosteroid and hyaluronic acid preparations, have been used as alternatives in such patients.

CORTICOSTEROIDS — Intra-articular corticosteroid injections, usually of methylprednisolone or triamcinolone, are preferred over intra-articular injections of other drugs for treatment of osteoarthritis pain. They can be effective even in joints that are not obviously inflamed.[26] Ideally, they should serve as a bridge to long-term interventions such as physical therapy, home exercises, weight management, and bracing. A 1-year, randomized trial in 156 patients with knee osteoarthritis compared glucocorticoid injections (mean of 2.6 injections) with physical therapy (mean of 11.8 treatment visits); pain and disability scores were lower with physical therapy.[27]

Efficacy – About 80% of patients with symptomatic osteoarthritis of the knee have a therapeutic response to intra-articular corticosteroid injections. Pain relief usually lasts for at least one month. The effect tends to wane by 2 months, but most clinicians wait a minimum of 3 months between injections. Mixing a local anesthetic such as lidocaine 1% with the corticosteroid can provide immediate pain relief and ensure the accuracy of the injection.

Adverse Effects – Intra-articular corticosteroid injections are generally safe. Some patients may develop a local inflammatory reaction. Septic arthritis is rare. Other uncommon local adverse effects include bleeding, tendinopathy, tendon rupture, lipoatrophy, skin atrophy, and avascular necrosis. In one randomized trial in 140 patients with knee osteoarthritis, there was significantly greater cartilage loss with intra-articular injections of triamcinolone 40 mg every 3 months for 2 years than with placebo injections and no significant difference in knee pain.[28]

Systemic effects are rare. Flushing can occur several hours after injection. Adverse effects commonly associated with systemic steroid use such as osteoporosis and gastric ulcers have not been reported with intra-articular injection of corticosteroids. In some patients with diabetes, intra-articular corticosteroids can increase blood glucose levels.

HYALURONIC ACID — Commercially available hyaluronic acid preparations injected into the joint space are claimed to increase the viscoelasticity of synovial fluid and possibly prevent degradation of articular cartilage. Intra-articular injections of hyaluronic acid are FDA-approved for osteoarthritis of the knee, but they have had only modest beneficial effects. ACR guidelines state that when meta-analysis is limited to trials with low risk of bias, the effect size of hyaluronic acid compared to saline injections approaches zero.[29] There are no reliable data showing that hyaluronic acid injections slow progression of osteoarthritis.

1. SL Kolasinski et al. 2019 American College of Rheumatology/Arthritis Foundation guideline for the management of osteoarthritis of the hand, hip, and knee. Arthritis Rheumatol 2020; 72:220.
2. S Wongrakpanich et al. A comprehensive review of non-steroidal anti-inflammatory drug use in the elderly. Aging Dis 2018; 9:143.

3. F Rannou et al. Efficacy and safety of topical NSAIDs in the management of osteoarthritis: evidence from real-life setting trials and surveys. Semin Arthritis Rheum 2016; 45(4 Suppl):S18.
4. FKL Chan et al. Gastrointestinal safety of celecoxib versus naproxen in patients with cardiothrombotic diseases and arthritis after upper gastrointestinal bleeding (CONCERN): an industry-independent, double-blind, double-dummy, randomised trial. Lancet 2017; 389:2375.
5. S Trelle et al. Cardiovascular safety of non-steroidal anti-inflammatory drugs: network meta-analysis. BMJ 2011; 342:c7086.
6. SE Nissen et al. Cardiovascular safety of celecoxib, naproxen, or ibuprofen for arthritis. N Engl J Med 2016; 375:2519.
7. Celecoxib safety revisited. Med Lett Drugs Ther 2016; 58:159.
8. Diclofenac gel for osteoarthritis. Med Lett Drugs Ther 2008; 50:31.
9. DK Li et al. Use of nonsteroidal antiinflammatory drugs during pregnancy and the risk of miscarriage. Am J Obstet Gynecol 2018; 219:275.
10. Inhibitors and inducers of CYP enzymes and P-glycoprotein. Med Lett Drugs Ther 2019 November 6 (epub). Available at: medicalletter.org/downloads/CYP_PGP_Tables.pdf.
11. BR da Costa et al. Effectiveness of non-steroidal anti-inflammatory drugs for the treatment of pain in knee and hip osteoarthritis: a network meta-analysis. Lancet 2017; 390:e21.
12. In brief: does acetaminophen increase blood pressure? Med Lett Drugs Ther 2011; 53:29.
13. Addendum: warfarin-acetaminophen interaction. Med Lett Drugs Ther 2008; 50:45.
14. S Karami et al. Analgesic use and risk of renal cell carcinoma: a case-control, cohort and meta-analytic assessment. Int J Cancer 2016; 139:584.
15. Z Liew et al. Acetaminophen use during pregnancy, behavioral problems, and hyperkinetic disorders. JAMA Pediatr 2014; 168:313.
16. Y Ji et al. Association of cord plasma biomarkers of in utero acetaminophen exposure with risk of attention-deficit/hyperactivity disorder and autism spectrum disorder in childhood. JAMA Psychiatry 2020; 77:180.
17. Duloxetine (Cymbalta) for chronic musculoskeletal pain. Med Lett Drugs Ther 2011; 53:33.
18. ZY Wang et al. Efficacy and safety of duloxetine on osteoarthritis knee pain: a meta-analysis of randomized controlled trials. Pain Med 2015; 16:1373.
19. JW Busse et al. Opioids for chronic noncancer pain: a systematic review and meta-analysis. JAMA 2018; 320:2448.
20. Opioids for pain. Med Lett Drugs Ther 2018; 60:57.
21. Another once-daily formulation of tramadol (Ryzolt). Med Lett Drugs Ther 2010; 52:39.
22. C Gabay et al. Symptomatic effects of chondroitin 4 and chondroitin 6 sulfate on hand osteoarthritis: a randomized, double-blind, placebo-controlled clinical trial at a single center. Arthritis Rheum 2011; 63:3383.
23. Turmeric supplements. Med Lett Drugs Ther 2019; 61:185.
24. TE McAlindon et al. OARSI guidelines for the non-surgical management of knee osteoarthritis. Osteoarthritis Cartilage 2014; 22:363.
25. RD Altman and HR Barthel. Topical therapies for osteoarthritis. Drugs 2011; 71:1259.
26. Two new intra-articular injections for knee osteoarthritis. Med Lett Drugs Ther 2018; 60:142.

27. GD Deyle et al. Physical therapy versus glucocorticoid injection for osteoarthritis of the knee. N Engl J Med 2020; 382:1420.

28. TE McAlindon et al. Effect of intra-articular triamcinolone vs saline on knee cartilage volume and pain in patients with knee osteoarthritis: a randomized clinical trial. JAMA 2017; 317:1967.

29. AW Rutjes et al. Viscosupplementation for osteoarthritis of the knee: a systematic review and meta-analysis. Ann Intern Med 2012; 157:180.

30. Z Wang et al. Effectiveness of Curcuma longa extract for the treatment of symptoms and effusion-synovitis of knee osteoarthritis: a randomized trial. Ann Intern Med 2020 September 15 (epub).

DRUGS FOR
Postmenopausal Osteoporosis

Original publication date – July 2020

US guidelines recommend pharmacologic therapy for postmenopausal women with a bone density T-score (standard deviation from normal mean values in healthy young women) of -2.5 or below in the lumbar spine, femoral neck, total hip, or distal radius, a T-score between -1.0 and -2.5 and a history of fragility (low-trauma) fracture of the hip or spine, or a T-score between -1.0 and -2.5 and a FRAX 10-year probability of ≥3% for hip fracture or ≥20% for major osteoporotic fracture (hip, clinical spine, humerus, distal radius).[1,2]

CALCIUM AND VITAMIN D

There is no convincing evidence that use of calcium and vitamin D supplements in addition to drugs for treatment of osteoporosis reduces fracture risk in postmenopausal women with osteoporosis, except for those living in nursing homes.[3,4] Nevertheless, calcium and vitamin D supplements are generally recommended for postmenopausal women with osteoporosis, and all recent trials of drugs for treatment of osteo-porosis include calcium and vitamin D supplements as the standard baseline treatment.

The Institute of Medicine recommends a calcium intake of 1000-1200 mg/day from diet (preferred) and/or supplements.[5] The 25-hydroxyvitamin D (25[OH]D) serum level of ≥30 ng/mL

209

Summary: Drugs for Postmenopausal Osteoporosis

▶ Postmenopausal women with osteoporosis should have an adequate calcium intake and take vitamin D supplements in addition to pharmacotherapy to reduce fracture risk.

▶ Bisphosphonates are antiresorptive agents that limit bone breakdown. The oral bisphosphonates alendronate (*Fosamax*, and others) and risedronate (*Actonel*, and others) and IV zoledronic acid (*Reclast*, and generics) can reduce the risk of vertebral and hip and other nonvertebral fractures. IV ibandronate (*Boniva*, and generics) has only been shown to reduce the risk of vertebral fractures.

▶ Denosumab (*Prolia*) is a subcutaneously injected antiresorptive drug that can reduce the risk of vertebral and hip and other nonvertebral fractures. It is an alternative to a bisphosphonate for patients at high risk for fracture or for those who have not responded to or cannot tolerate bisphosphonates.

▶ The parathyroid hormone analogs teriparatide (*Forteo*, and generics) and abaloparatide (*Tymlos*) are anabolic agents that can increase bone mineral density and reduce the risk of vertebral and nonvertebral fractures, but they must be injected daily and should only be used for a maximum of 2 years in the patient's lifetime.

▶ The selective estrogen receptor modulator (SERM) raloxifene (*Evista*, and generics) can increase bone mineral density and has been shown to reduce the risk of vertebral fractures, but not nonvertebral fractures. It is recommended for use in women at high risk for invasive breast cancer.

▶ A fixed-dose combination of the SERM bazedoxifene and conjugated estrogens (*Duavee*) can prevent osteoporosis and reduce vasomotor symptoms; it should not be used solely for prevention or treatment of osteoporosis.

▶ The anabolic sclerostin inhibitor romosozumab (*Evenity*) stimulates bone formation and decreases bone resorption. In clinical trials, it was more effective than alendronate in reducing vertebral and clinical fractures and more effective than teriparatide in increasing hip bone mineral density. It could be considered for initial treatment of women at very high risk of fracture.

recommended by the American Society of Clinical Endocrinologists (AACE) and the Endocrine Society can generally be achieved by taking a daily supplement of 1000-2000 IU of vitamin D.

Products – Calcium carbonate should be taken with food to enhance absorption. Calcium citrate does not require acid for absorption and can

Table 1. Diagnosis of Osteoporosis in Postmenopausal Women[1]
- T-score of -2.5 or below in the lumbar spine, femoral neck, total hip, or distal radius
- Low-trauma spine or hip fracture, regardless of bone mineral density
- T-score between -1.0 and -2.5 and a fragility fracture of the proximal humerus, pelvis, or distal forearm
- T-score between -1.0 and -2.5 and a FRAX 10-year probability of ≥3% for hip fracture or ≥20% for major osteoporotic fracture

1. PM Camacho et al. Endocr Pract 2020; 26(Suppl 1):1.

be taken with or without food; it is preferred for patients taking a proton pump inhibitor (PPI) or an H_2-receptor antagonist. Other calcium salts can be taken without regard to food.

Vitamin D supplements are available as ergocalciferol (vitamin D_2) or cholecalciferol (vitamin D_3); vitamin D_3 increases 25(OH)D levels more than vitamin D_2 and is preferred.

Adverse Effects – Calcium supplements are generally well tolerated, but they can cause constipation, intestinal bloating, and excess gas. Doses ≥1000 mg/day have been associated with an increased risk of nephrolithiasis.[6]

Some reports have suggested that calcium supplementation could increase the risk of myocardial infarction,[7] but in the Women's Health Initiative trial, among 36,282 postmenopausal women randomized to receive either calcium (1000 mg/day) plus vitamin D_3 (400 IU/day) or placebo, 7 years of calcium plus vitamin D supplementation did not increase the incidence of coronary heart disease, myocardial infarction, or stroke.[8] A systematic review found that a daily calcium intake of 2000-2500 mg was not associated with an increased risk of cardiovascular disease in generally healthy adults.[9]

Hypercalcemia and hypercalciuria can occur with high doses of vitamin D.

BISPHOSPHONATES

These nonhormonal drugs decrease bone resorption by binding to active sites of bone remodeling and inhibiting osteoclasts. Alendronate, risedronate, and zoledronic acid have been shown to reduce the risk of vertebral and hip and other nonvertebral fractures in postmenopausal women; ibandronate has only been shown to reduce the risk of vertebral fractures.

ALENDRONATE — Oral alendronate (*Fosamax*, and others) is FDA-approved for prevention and treatment of osteoporosis in postmenopausal women. Once-weekly dosing appears to be as effective as daily dosing in increasing bone mineral density (BMD) and may be better tolerated.

IBANDRONATE — Oral ibandronate (*Boniva*, and generics) taken once a month is FDA-approved for prevention and treatment of postmenopausal osteoporosis. IV ibandronate administered once every three months is only approved for treatment; it appears to be more effective than the oral formulation in increasing BMD.[10]

RISEDRONATE — Oral risedronate (*Actonel*, and others) is FDA-approved for prevention and treatment of osteoporosis in postmenopausal women. Once-weekly and once-monthly regimens appear to have similar effects on BMD.

ZOLEDRONIC ACID — IV zoledronic acid (*Reclast*, and generics) is FDA-approved for treatment (once yearly) and prevention (once every two years) of osteoporosis in postmenopausal women.

ORAL ADMINISTRATION — Food, calcium supplements, antacids, and other drugs containing polyvalent cations, such as iron, interfere with the absorption of bisphosphonates from the GI tract. To ensure adequate absorption and prevent esophageal injury, oral bisphosphonates must be taken after an overnight fast, while in an upright position, with 6-8 ounces of plain (not mineral) water. After taking the drug, patients should not consume anything by mouth except plain water for at least 30 minutes

Table 2. Calcium Content of Some Foods[1]

Food[2]	Serving Size	Calcium (mg)[3]
Breakfast cereals[4]	1 cup	130
Broccoli, raw	1 cup	42
Cheese, cheddar, reduced fat	1.5 oz	307
Cheese, mozzarella, part-skim	1.5 oz	333
Cheese, provolone	1 slice	212
Cheese, swiss	1 slice	200
Cottage cheese, 1% fat	1 cup	138
Kale, cooked	1 cup	94
Milk, soy (calcium-fortified)	1 cup	299
Milk, skim	1 cup	299
Oatmeal, instant (regular)	1 packet	21
Orange juice (calcium-fortified)	1 cup	349
Spinach, boiled	1/2 cup	40
Tofu, raw, firm	1/2 cup	138
Yogurt, plain	8 oz	415

1. US Department of Agriculture. Food data central. Available at: https://fdc.nal.usda.gov. Accessed July 2, 2020.
2. Some foods, such as spinach, contain oxalic acid, which may limit the absorption of calcium.
3. Approximate content per serving.
4. Calcium content of cereals varies; *Total Whole Grain* cereal (General Mills) contains 1000 mg of calcium per 3/4 cup serving.

(60 minutes for ibandronate) and remain upright for 30-60 minutes. The enteric-coated, delayed-release, once-weekly formulation of risedronate (*Atelvia*, and generics) can be taken immediately after breakfast with at least 4 ounces of plain water.

ADVERSE EFFECTS — Oral bisphosphonates can cause heartburn, esophageal irritation, esophagitis, abdominal pain, diarrhea, and other GI adverse effects. Acute-phase reactions (low-grade fevers, myalgias, and arthralgias) have been reported. Severe bone, joint, and muscle pain has occurred infrequently. Ocular inflammation has also been reported. Hypocalcemia can occur, typically in patients with vitamin D deficiency.

IV bisphosphonates have also been associated with acute-phase reactions within 1-3 days of the infusion, most frequently after the first infusion; an

Table 3. Vitamin D Content of Some Foods[1]		
Food[2]	Serving Size	Vitamin D (IU)[3]
Egg, whole large	1 egg	50
Milk, skim (fortified)	1 cup	120
Milk, soy (fortified)	8 oz	104
Milk, whole (fortified)	1 cup	96
Mushrooms (white)	1/2 cup	366
Salmon, sockeye, cooked	3 oz	570
Sardines, canned	1 cup	288
Trout (rainbow)	3 oz	645
Tuna, light, canned	3 oz	40

1. US Department of Agriculture. Food data central. Available at: https://fdc.nal.usda.gov. Accessed July 2, 2020.
2. Many other products, including breakfast cereals and margarine, are often fortified with vitamin D.
3. Approximate content per serving.

NSAID or acetaminophen can decrease the severity of symptoms. Renal failure and death have occurred in patients with renal impairment (creatinine clearance <35 mL/min) treated with IV zoledronic acid; the drug is contraindicated for use in such patients.[11]

Osteonecrosis of the jaw (ONJ) has occurred rarely (1/50,000 osteoporosis patients) with chronic use of oral bisphosphonates. The incidence of ONJ has been higher in patients with cancer or immunosuppression treated with high-dose IV bisphosphonates. Other risk factors include denosumab use, dental extractions, and periodontal infection.[12]

Atypical femoral fractures have been reported with use of bisphosphonates. The absolute risk of these fractures is low, ranging from 3.2 to 50 cases per 100,000 person-years; the risk increases with long-term use (~100 cases per 100,000 person-years).[13] Among >52,000 women taking a bisphosphonate for at least 5 years, an atypical subtrochanteric or femoral shaft fracture occurred during the subsequent year in 0.13% of women and within 2 years in 0.22%.[14]

DURATION OF TREATMENT — The optimal duration of treatment with bisphosphonates is unclear. Among 1099 postmenopausal women who had received alendronate for 5 years and were randomized to receive an additional 5 years of alendronate or placebo, those who remained on alendronate had a significantly lower risk of developing clinically recognized vertebral fractures (2.4% vs 5.3%), but not nonvertebral fractures; women considered to be at high risk for fracture, based on low total hip BMD, were excluded from the trial.[15] Because of the association between long-term bisphosphonate use and atypical femoral fractures, some experts discontinue bisphosphonates temporarily after 5 years of oral use (or 3 years of IV administration) in patients at low risk for fracture (stable bone density, femoral neck T-score of -2.5 or higher, no history of hip or spine fracture). When to restart these drugs in such patients is unclear.

DENOSUMAB

Denosumab *(Prolia)* is a fully humanized anti-RANK ligand monoclonal antibody that inhibits osteoclast formation, function, and survival, thereby reducing bone resorption. It is FDA-approved for treatment of osteoporosis in postmenopausal women at high risk for fracture (history of osteoporotic fracture or multiple risk factors for fracture) and is an alternative in patients who have not responded to or cannot tolerate bisphosphonates.

Injected subcutaneously once every 6 months, denosumab has been shown to increase BMD and reduce the incidence of new vertebral and hip and other nonvertebral fractures in postmenopausal women. It has been shown to increase BMD more than alendronate, but no large randomized trials directly comparing denosumab with bisphosphonates for prevention of fractures are available. In a nationwide Danish population-based cohort study, the risks of hip or any fracture over a 3-year period were similar with denosumab and alendronate.[16]

DURATION OF TREATMENT — The optimal duration of treatment with denosumab is unclear. Available data support its continued efficacy for 10 years.[17] The effects of denosumab on BMD and bone turnover are reversible when the drug is stopped. Stopping the drug after 24 months of treatment resulted in increased bone turnover markers within 3 months and a decline in BMD to pretreatment values within 2 years.[18] Vertebral fractures have been reported 8-16 months after stopping denosumab.[19] Drug holidays are not recommended. If denosumab is stopped, starting another drug, typically a bisphosphonate, is recommended to prevent a rapid decline in BMD. Switching from denosumab to teriparatide has resulted in bone loss.[20]

ADVERSE EFFECTS — Denosumab can cause hypocalcemia, especially in patients with renal impairment. In clinical trials, rash, eczema, and dermatitis occurred more commonly with denosumab than with placebo. Osteonecrosis of the jaw and atypical femoral fractures, which can occur with bisphosphonates, have also been reported with denosumab, but not at higher-than-background rates in age-matched populations.

PARATHYROID HORMONE ANALOGS

Daily subcutaneous injection of parathyroid hormone (PTH) or parathyroid hormone-related protein (PTHrP) analogs increases BMD by stimulating bone formation. They are recommended for treatment of osteoporosis in postmenopausal women who are at high risk for fracture or have not responded to or cannot tolerate other available osteoporosis therapies. **Teriparatide** (*Forteo*, and others), the recombinant 1-34 sequence of human PTH, and **abaloparatide** *(Tymlos)*, a synthetic analog of human parathyroid hormone-related peptide, are FDA-approved for treatment of osteoporosis for up to 2 years in the patient's lifetime in postmenopausal women at high risk for fracture. A bisphosphonate or denosumab should be started after stopping these drugs.

TERIPARATIDE — Once-daily injections of teriparatide have been shown to increase BMD at the lumbar spine, femoral neck, and hip and decrease the incidence of vertebral and nonvertebral fractures by 50% or more compared to risedronate.[21] BMD decreases after the drug is stopped, but retreatment after a drug-free period has been shown to produce small gains in BMD.[22,23] Switching from teriparatide or a combination of

Table 4. Some Calcium and Vitamin D Supplements		
Drug	Ca (mg)[1]	D₃ (IU)[1]
Calcium Carbonate[2]		
Caltrate 600+D₃ (Pfizer)	600	800
Os-Cal Calcium + D₃ (GSK)	500	200
Tums Extra Strength 750 (GSK)	300	—
Viactiv Calcium plus D (Viactiv Lifestyle)[3]	500	500
Calcium Citrate[2]		
Citracal Maximum Plus (Bayer)	325	500
Citracal Petites (Bayer)	200	250
Calcium Complex (carbonate, lactate)		
Calcet Petites (MainPointe)	200	250
Calcium Phosphate[2]		
Citracal Calcium Gummies (Bayer)[4]	250	500
Posture-D (International Vitamin Corp)[5]	600	500

1. Elemental calcium and vitamin D content per tablet.
2. Also available generically.
3. Content of milk chocolate and caramel soft chews; also contains 40 mcg vitamin K.
4. Also contains 107 mg phosphorus.
5. Also contains 280 mg phosphorus and 50 mg magnesium.

teriparatide and denosumab to denosumab monotherapy results in further increases in BMD.[20]

ABALOPARATIDE — In a randomized, double-blind, 18-month trial (ACTIVE) in 2463 postmenopausal women with osteoporosis, 63% of whom had a history of fracture, once-daily injections of abaloparatide significantly increased BMD at the hip, femoral neck, and lumbar spine and reduced the rate of new vertebral fractures (0.6% vs 4.2% with placebo). The Kaplan-Meier estimated rate of nonvertebral fractures was also significantly lower with abaloparatide than with placebo (2.7% vs 4.7%).[24]

Abaloparatide also appears to produce greater increases in BMD than teriparatide, but not significantly greater decreases in the incidence of

Table 5. Some Drugs for Postmenopausal Osteoporosis

Drug	Some Formulations
Bisphosphonates	
Alendronate – generic	5, 10, 35, 70 mg tabs; 70 mg/75 mL oral soln
Fosamax (Merck)	70 mg tabs
Fosamax Plus D	70 mg/2800 IU D_3, 70 mg/5600 IU D_3 tabs
Binosto (Ascend)	70 mg effervescent tabs
Ibandronate – generic	150 mg tabs; 3 mg/3 mL prefilled syringes and vials
Boniva (Genentech)	150 mg tabs; 3 mg/3 mL prefilled syringes
Risedronate – generic *Actonel* (Allergan)	5, 35, 150 mg tabs[6]
delayed-release – generic *Atelvia* (Allergan)	35 mg delayed-release tabs
Zoledronic acid[7] – generic *Reclast* (Novartis)	5 mg/100 mL IV soln
Anti-RANK Ligand Antibody	
Denosumab – *Prolia* (Amgen)[9]	60 mg/mL prefilled syringes
Parathyroid Hormone Analogs	
Abaloparatide – *Tymlos* (Radius)[11]	3120 mcg/1.56 mL prefilled pens
Teriparatide – generic *Forteo* (Lilly)	600 mcg/2.4 mL prefilled pens
Selective Estrogen Receptor Modulator	
Raloxifene – generic *Evista* (Lilly)	60 mg tabs

1. Dosage adjustments may be needed for renal or hepatic impairment.
2. Approximate WAC for 30 days' treatment at the lowest usual adult dosage or frequency. Cost of *Duavee* is based on dosage used for prevention. WAC = wholesaler acquisition cost or manufacturer's published price to wholesalers; WAC represents a published catalogue or list price and may not represent an actual transactional price. Source: AnalySource® Monthly. June 5, 2020. Reprinted with permission by First Databank, Inc. All rights reserved. ©2020. www.fdbhealth.com/policies/drug-pricing-policy.
3. Should be dissolved in 4 oz of room-temperature plain water.
4. Cost for tablets. Cost of one generic 3 mg/mL syringe is $240.00.
5. Cost of one syringe.

Usual Adult Dosage[1]	Cost[2]
Prevention: 5 mg PO once/day or 35 mg once/wk	$21.10
Treatment: 10 mg PO once/day or 70 mg once/wk	127.80
Treatment: 70 mg/2800 IU D$_3$ or 70 mg/5600 IU D$_3$ PO once/wk	173.30
Treatment: 70 mg PO once/wk[3]	300.00
Prevention: 150 mg PO once/mo	10.00[4]
Treatment: 150 mg PO once/mo or 3 mg IV once every 3 mos	527.40[5]
Prevention: 5 mg PO once/day, 35 mg once/wk, or 150 mg once/mo	166.00
	369.30
Treatment: 5 mg PO once/day, 35 mg once/wk, 75 mg 2 consecutive days/mo, or 150 mg once/mo	
Treatment: 35 mg PO once/wk	171.60
	266.60
Prevention: 5 mg IV once every 2 years	235.00[8]
Treatment: 5 mg IV once/year	1083.80[8]
Treatment: 60 mg SC once every 6 mos	1278.80[10]
Treatment: 80 mcg SC once/day[12]	1966.40[10]
Treatment: 20 mcg SC once/day[12]	2475.00[10]
	3597.80[10]
Prevention: 60 mg PO once/day	60.00
Treatment: 60 mg PO once/day	198.00

6. Risedronate is also available in a 30-mg tablet for treatment of Paget's disease.
7. Zoledronic acid is also available in a 4-mg formulation (*Zometa*, and generics) for treatment of hypercalcemia of malignancy, multiple myeloma, and bone metastases from solid tumors.
8. Cost of one 5 mg/100 mL infusion bottle.
9. Denosumab is also available in a 120 mg/1.7 mL formulation (*Xgeva*) for prevention of skeletal-related events in patients with bone metastases from solid tumors.
10. Cost of one syringe or prefilled pen.
11. Abaloparatide is a parathyroid hormone-related protein analog.
12. Cumulative use for more than 2 years during a patient's lifetime is not recommended.

Continued on next page

Drugs for Postmenopausal Osteoporosis

Table 5. Some Drugs for Postmenopausal Osteoporosis (continued)	
Drug	**Some Formulations**
Conjugated Estrogens and Selective Estrogen Receptor Modulator[13]	
Conjugated estrogens and bazedoxifene – *Duavee* (Pfizer)	0.45 mg/20 mg tabs
Sclerostin Inhibitor	
Romosozumab-aqqg – *Evenity* (Amgen)	105 mg/1.17 mL prefilled syringes
Calcitonin[14]	
Calcitonin – generic	200 IU/spray

13. Conjugated estrogens are no longer recommended for first-line treatment of postmenopausal osteoporosis because of an increased risk of breast cancer, stroke, and venous thromboembolism.
14. Because of safety concerns and limited evidence of efficacy, many experts no longer recommend use of salmon calcitonin.

fractures.[25] Unlike teriparatide, it does not have to be refrigerated after first use.

ADVERSE EFFECTS — Teriparatide can cause nausea, arthralgia, and pain. Hypotension and tachycardia may occur with the first few doses. Transient hypercalcemia and hypercalciuria can occur; they can generally be corrected by reducing calcium intake. Teriparatide should not be used in patients with pre-existing hypercalcemia, bone metastases, or skeletal malignancies. The labeling of teriparatide includes a boxed warning about a risk of osteosarcoma based on animal data, but in a postmarketing surveillance study, none of the 1448 cases of osteosarcoma identified in the US in a 7-year period were associated with use of teriparatide.[26]

Abaloparatide can cause injection-site reactions, dizziness, nausea, headache, palpitations, tachycardia, orthostatic hypotension, hypercalcemia, hypercalciuria, and hyperuricemia. In one trial, the incidence of adverse events leading to discontinuation was higher with abaloparatide (9.9%) than with teriparatide (6.8%) or placebo (6.1%).[27] As with teriparatide, the labeling of abaloparatide includes a boxed warning about a risk of osteosarcoma based on animal data.

Usual Adult Dosage[1]	Cost[2]
Prevention: 0.45 mg/20 mg PO once/day	$185.60
Treatment: 210 mg SC once/mo x 12 doses	1825.00
Treatment: 200 IU intranasally once/day	74.90[15]

15. Cost of one 3.7-mL bottle.

SELECTIVE ESTROGEN RECEPTOR MODULATORS

RALOXIFENE — Raloxifene (*Evista*, and generics), a selective estrogen receptor modulator (SERM) with estrogen-like effects on bone and anti-estrogen effects on the uterus and breast, is FDA-approved for prevention and treatment of postmenopausal osteoporosis. It has reduced the risk of vertebral fractures, but not nonvertebral fractures.[28] Raloxifene can reduce the risk of invasive breast cancer and may be a reasonable alternative to bisphosphonate therapy in postmenopausal women at high risk for invasive breast cancer. Bisphosphonates are generally preferred over raloxifene for **treatment** of osteoporosis in postmenopausal women because they are more effective in preventing nonvertebral and hip fractures.[29]

Adverse Effects – Hot flashes, leg cramps, and peripheral edema can occur with raloxifene. Like estrogens, raloxifene increases the risk of venous thromboembolic events.

CONJUGATED ESTROGENS/BAZEDOXIFENE — A fixed-dose combination of the SERM bazedoxifene and conjugated estrogens *(Duavee)* is FDA-approved for prevention of osteoporosis and treatment of vasomotor symptoms in postmenopausal women with an intact uterus.

Table 6. Fracture Risk Reduction by Site[1,2]

Drug	Vertebral Fractures	Nonvertebral Fractures	Hip Fractures
Bisphosphonates			
Alendronate (*Fosamax*, and others)	Yes	Yes	Yes
Ibandronate (*Boniva*, and generics)	Yes	No	No
Risedronate (*Actonel*, and others)	Yes	Yes	Yes
Zoledronic acid (*Reclast*, and generics)	Yes	Yes	Yes
Anti-RANK Ligand Antibody			
Denosumab (*Prolia*, and generics)	Yes	Yes	Yes
Parathyroid Hormone Analogs			
Abaloparatide *(Tymlos)*	Yes	Yes	No
Teriparatide (*Forteo*, and generics)	Yes	Yes	No
Selective Estrogen Receptor Modulator			
Raloxifene (*Evista*, and generics)	Yes	No	No
Conjugated Estrogens/Selective Estrogen Receptor Modulator			
Conjugated estrogens/ bazedoxifene *(Duavee)*	Yes	No	No
Sclerostin Inhibitor			
Romosozumab-aqqg *(Evenity)*	Yes	Yes[3]	Yes[3]
Calcitonin			
Calcitonin nasal[4]	Yes	No	No

1. PM Camacho et al. Endocr Pract 2020; 26(Suppl 1):1.
2. Trials may not have been adequately powered to demonstrate fracture risk reduction at these sites.
3. In the ARCH trial, 12 months' treatment with romosozumab followed by alendronate for 12 months reduced nonvertebral and hip fractures compared to 24 months' treatment with alendronate. K Saag et al. N Engl J Med 2017; 277:1417.
4. No published studies are available demonstrating the efficacy of injectable calcitonin for fracture prevention.

It should not be used solely for prevention or treatment of osteoporosis. The combination has been shown to increase BMD in postmenopausal women, and bazedoxifene alone (not available commercially) has been shown to decrease the risk of vertebral fractures.[30,31] Like raloxifene, bazedoxifene inhibits the stimulating effect of estrogen on the endometrium and breast. Unlike raloxifene, bazedoxifene has not been shown to reduce the risk of breast cancer.

Adverse Effects – Muscle spasms, nausea, dyspepsia, and abdominal, neck, and oropharyngeal pain have been reported with use of the combination. In short-term clinical trials of conjugated estrogens/bazedoxifene, the combination did not increase the incidence of breast cancer, endometrial cancer, ovarian cancer, venous thromboembolism (VTE), stroke, myocardial infarction, or death from any cause. The long-term safety of the combination remains to be determined. In a randomized, double-blind trial in postmenopausal women with osteoporosis, venous thromboembolic events, primarily deep vein thrombosis (DVT), occurred more frequently in women taking bazedoxifene alone for 5 years than in those taking placebo.[32]

ROMOSOZUMAB

Romosozumab *(Evenity)* is a monoclonal antibody that binds to and inhibits sclerostin, increasing bone formation and decreasing bone resorption.[33,34] It is FDA-approved for once-monthly subcutaneous treatment of osteoporosis for up to one year in postmenopausal women who are at high risk for fracture or have not responded to or could not tolerate other drugs for this indication.

In one trial (FRAME), 7180 postmenopausal women with osteoporosis and a T-score of -2.5 to -3.5 in the total hip or femoral neck were randomized to receive romosozumab or placebo for 12 months; both groups then received denosumab for an additional 12 months. At 12 months, new vertebral fractures had occurred in 0.5% of women receiving romosozumab and in 1.8% of those receiving placebo, a statistically significant difference. There was no significant difference between the groups in the occurrence of nonvertebral fractures. At 24 months, after both groups had switched to denosumab, the vertebral fracture rate was still significantly lower in the group originally treated with romosozumab (0.6% vs 2.5%).[35]

In an active-comparator trial (ARCH) in 4093 postmenopausal women with osteoporosis and a fragility fracture, patients randomized to receive romosozumab for 12 months followed by alendronate for an additional 12 months had a 48% lower risk of new vertebral fractures, a 19% lower risk of nonvertebral fractures, and a 38% lower risk of hip fracture after an average of 33 months compared to those who received alendronate for 12 months followed by open-label alendronate.[36]

In a randomized, double-blind, active-controlled trial (STRUCTURE), 436 postmenopausal women with osteoporosis who had taken an oral bisphosphonate for ≥3 years and alendronate within the past year and had a T-score of -2.5 or lower at the total hip, femoral neck, or lumbar spine and a history of fracture were randomized to receive romosozumab 210 mg SC once monthly or teriparatide 20 mcg SC once daily. The mean change from baseline in BMD at the total hip at 12 months, the primary endpoint, was 2.6% with romosozumab and -0.6% with teriparatide, a statistically significant difference.[37]

ADVERSE EFFECTS — Arthralgia and headache were the most common adverse effects reported with use of romosozumab in clinical trials. In FRAME and ARCH, 3 atypical femoral fractures and 3 cases of jaw osteonecrosis were reported in patients who received romosozumab. Serious adverse cardiovascular events occurred more frequently with romosozumab than with alendronate in ARCH (2.5% vs 1.9%); the rate in FRAME was not higher with romosozumab than with placebo. Romosozumab should not be used in patients who had a myocardial infarction or stroke within the previous year. Neutralizing antibodies to romosozumab have developed; whether they reduce the efficacy of the drug is unknown.

CALCITONIN

Salmon calcitonin is FDA-approved for treatment of osteoporosis in women >5 years after menopause when alternative treatments are not suitable. It decreases bone resorption by inhibiting osteoclast function. A 5-year trial in women with osteoporosis found new vertebral fractures in 51 of 287 (18%) receiving a 200-IU dose of calcitonin nasal spray once daily and in 70 of 270 (26%) receiving a placebo, a statistically significant difference.[38]

ADVERSE EFFECTS — Serious allergic reactions, including anaphylaxis, have occurred with use of calcitonin. An increased risk of malignancy has been reported with use of calcitonin nasal spray.[39,40]

Given the limited evidence of its efficacy, concerns about its safety, and the availability of other options, many expert clinicians no longer recommend calcitonin. It has been removed from the market in Canada and Europe.

1. PM Camacho et al. American Association of Clinical Endocrinologists/American College of Endocrinology clinical practice guidelines for the diagnosis and treatment of postmenopausal osteoporosis – 2020 update. Endocr Pract 2020; 26(Suppl 1):1.
2. FRAX. Fracture risk assessment tool. Available at www.sheffield.ac.uk/FRAX/tool.aspx-?country=9. Accessed July 1, 2020.
3. US Preventive Services Task Force. Vitamin D, calcium, or combined supplementation for the primary prevention of fractures in community-dwelling adults: US Preventive Services Task Force recommendation statement. JAMA 2018; 319:1592.
4. IR Reid and MJ Bolland. Controversies in medicine: the role of calcium and vitamin D supplements in adults. Med J Aust 2019; 211:468.
5. AC Ross et al. The 2011 report on dietary reference intakes for calcium and vitamin D from the Institute of Medicine: what clinicians need to know. J Clin Endocrinol Metab 2011; 96:53.
6. RB Wallace et al. Urinary tract stone occurrence in the Women's Health Initiative (WHI) randomized clinical trial of calcium and vitamin D supplements. Am J Clin Nutr 2011; 94:270.
7. IR Reid. Cardiovascular effects of calcium supplements. Nutrients 2013; 5:2522.
8. RL Prentice et al. Health risks and benefits from calcium and vitamin D supplementation: Women's Health Initiative clinical trial and cohort study. Osteoporos Int 2013; 24:567.
9. M Chung et al. Calcium intake and cardiovascular disease risk: an updated systematic review and meta-analysis. Ann Intern Med 2016; 165:856.

10. JA Eisman et al. Efficacy and tolerability of intravenous ibandronate injections in postmenopausal osteoporosis: 2-year results from the DIVA study. J Rheumatol 2008; 35:488.

11. FDA drug safety communication: new contraindication and updated warning on kidney impairment for Reclast (zoledronic acid). Available at www.fda.gov/Drugs/DrugSafety/ucm270199.htm. Accessed July 1, 2020.

12. AA Khan et al. Case-based review of osteonecrosis of the jaw (ONJ) and application of the International Recommendations for Management from the International Task Force on ONJ. J Clin Densitom 2017; 20:8.

13. J Schilcher et al. Bisphosphonate use and atypical fractures of the femoral shaft. N Engl J Med 2011; 364:1728.

14. LY Park-Wyllie et al. Bisphosphonate use and the risk of subtrochanteric or femoral shaft fractures in older women. JAMA 2011; 305:783.

15. DM Black et al. Effects of continuing or stopping alendronate after 5 years of treatment: the Fracture Intervention Trial Long-term Extension (FLEX): a randomized trial. JAMA 2006; 296:2927.

16. AB Pedersen et al. Comparison of risk of osteoporotic fracture in denosumab vs alendronate treatment within 3 years of initiation. JAMA Netw Open 2019; 2:e192416.

17. HG Bone et al. 10 years of denosumab treatment in postmenopausal women with osteoporosis: results from the phase 3 randomised FREEDOM trial and open-label extension. Lancet Diabetes Endocrinol 2017; 5:513.

18. HG Bone et al. Effects of denosumab treatment and discontinuation on bone mineral density and bone turnover markers in postmenopausal women with low bone mass. J Clin Endocrinol Metab 2011; 96:972.

19. AD Anastasilakis et al. Clinical features of 24 patients with rebound-associated vertebral fractures after denosumab discontinuation: systematic review and additional cases. J Bone Miner Res 2017; 32:1291.

20. BZ Leder et al. Denosumab and teriparatide transitions in postmenopausal osteoporosis (the DATA-Switch study): extension of a randomised controlled trial. Lancet 2015; 386:1147.

21. DL Kendler et al. Effects of teriparatide and risedronate on new fractures in postmenopausal women with severe osteoporosis (VERO): a multicentre, double-blind, double-dummy, randomised controlled trial. Lancet 2018; 391:230.

22. Teriparatide (Forteo) for osteoporosis. Med Lett Drugs Ther 2003; 45:9.

23. JS Finkelstein et al. Effects of teriparatide retreatment in osteoporotic men and women. J Clin Endocrinol Metab 2009; 94:2495.

24. Abaloparatide (Tymlos) for postmenopausal osteoporosis. Med Lett Drugs Ther 2017; 59:97.

25. PD Miller et al. Bone mineral density response rates are greater in patients treated with abaloparatide compared with those treated with placebo or teriparatide: results from the ACTIVE phase 3 trial. Bone 2019; 120:137.

26. EB Andrews et al. The US postmarketing surveillance study of adult osteosarcoma and teriparatide: study design and findings from the first 7 years. J Bone Miner Res 2012; 27:2429.

27. PD Miller et al. Effect of abaloparatide vs. placebo on new vertebral fractures in postmenopausal women with osteoporosis: a randomized clinical trial. JAMA 2016; 316:722.

28. KE Ensrud et al. Effects of raloxifene on fracture risk in postmenopausal women: the raloxifene use for the heart trial. J Bone Miner Res 2008; 23:112.
29. CJ Crandall et al. Comparative effectiveness of pharmacologic treatments to prevent fractures: an updated systematic review. Ann Intern Med 2014; 161:711.
30. Conjugated estrogens/bazedoxifene (Duavee) for menopausal symptoms and prevention of osteoporosis. Med Lett Drugs Ther 2014; 56:33.
31. JV Pinkerton et al. Effects of bazedoxifene/conjugated estrogens on the endometrium and bone: a randomized trial. J Clin Endocrinol Metab 2014; 99:e189.
32. TJ de Villiers et al. Safety and tolerability of bazedoxifene in postmenopausal women with osteoporosis: results of a 5-year, randomized, placebo-controlled phase 3 trial. Osteoporos Int 2011; 22:567.
33. Romosozumab (Evenity) for postmenopausal osteoporosis. Med Lett Drugs Ther 2019; 61:83.
34. D Shoback et al. Pharmacological management of osteoporosis in postmenopausal women: an Endocrine Society guideline update. J Clin Endocrinol Metab 2020; 105:587.
35. F Cosman et al. Romosozumab treatment in postmenopausal women with osteoporosis. N Engl J Med 2016; 375:1532.
36. KG Saag et al. Romosozumab or alendronate for fracture prevention in women with osteoporosis. N Engl J Med 2017; 377:1417.
37. BL Langdahl et al. Romosozumab (sclerostin monoclonal antibody) versus teriparatide in postmenopausal women with osteoporosis transitioning from oral bisphosphonate therapy: a randomised, open-label, phase 3 trial. Lancet 2017; 390:1585.
38. JA Knopp-Sihota et al. Calcitonin for treating acute and chronic pain of recent and remote osteoporotic vertebral compression fractures: a systematic review and meta-analysis. Osteoporos Int 2012; 23:17.
39. In brief: Cancer risk with salmon calcitonin. Med Lett Drugs Ther 2013; 55:29.
40. LM Sun et al. Calcitonin nasal spray and increased cancer risk: a population-based nested case-control study. J Clin Endocrinol Metab 2014; 99:4259.

Index

Index

Index

Index

Index